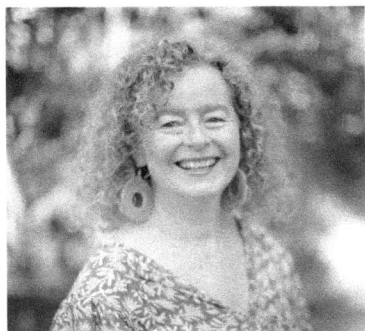

Sarah Jones and Ross, her husband of 32 years, live with their four adult children on Sydney's beautiful Northern Beaches. Sarah has a Diploma of Teaching (Primary) and has been a keen student of theology and history, among other things. Combining her passions for travel, photography and writing, Sarah has authored a travel blog over the past fourteen years, recounting family holidays and adventures. The blog has gained an avid readership.

Sarah also loves – in no particular order and sometimes simultaneously – live music, dancing, reality TV, cooking, reading, singing and the beach.

Sarah's mother, Jeannie Somerville, was diagnosed with dementia in 2014. It was this diagnosis, coupled with the lack of resources and reading material available for those undergoing similar experiences with loved ones, that prompted Sarah to write about her own journey with her mother's dementia, in the hope that it would help others.

This is Sarah's first book.

www.wordsbysarahjones.com

DEMENTIA, WHO ARE YOU AND WHAT HAVE YOU DONE WITH MY MOTHER?

Sarah Jones

First published in Australia in 2024 by Sarah Jones
thejonescrew6@icloud.com

A catalogue record for this
work is available from the
National Library of Australia

ISBN: 978 0 6458440 4 7 (Paperback)
ISBN: 978 0 6458440 5 4 (Ebook)

Produced by Broadcast Books, www.broadcastbooks.com.au
Edited by Bernadette Foley and Sophie Bellotti
Proofread by Puddingburn Publishing Services
Cover and text design by Liz Seymour, Seymour Design
Typeset in Garamond Premier Pro 12/18pt by Seymour Design
Author photograph by Sam Jones
Print and ebook by Ingram Spark

Some names have been changed to protect the identity of the individuals and institutions in question.

FOR SAM, MOLLY, TOBY AND MAISY

FOREWORDS

Sarah brings humour and insight to an experience tragically close to many people's hearts. She lays bare the trauma of dementia, as first her beloved mother Jeannie is diagnosed and then succumbs to its ever-greedier stages.

While Jeannie is robbed of almost everything for which she was known, Sarah never loses her way, detailing with honesty and love her mother's decline and the emotional fallout for the entire family. Sarah's narrative is raw and at times confronting but it is also warm and always engaging, as she candidly describes her struggles to navigate this confounding disease.

Sadly, Jeannie's illness stole her future. Sarah's devotion enshrined her mother's past, ensuring Jeannie will always be remembered for who she was, not for what she lost.

Tara Brown
Reporter, *60 Minutes*

This is the poignant and sensitive story of a daughter's love for her mother, Jeannie, who gradually develops dementia. It is an accurate and honest account of Sarah's mother's decline both mentally and physically, exploring the impact on Sarah's own family and those around her. It is a book that really tugs at one's heart strings, taking you deep inside the emotions of a daughter and her family as she deals with her mother's illness. It gives the reader a true insight into the tragedy that families face when dementia strikes.

Dr Tim Harpur
Jeannie Somerville's treating GP

PROLOGUE

The air was warm and thick with the scent of frangipanis; cicadas were singing their deafening tune. The kids were splashing around in the backyard pool and the early news had just come on the TV. This was my favourite time of year.

Wondering what on earth I had in the fridge that could possibly be fashioned into something edible, let alone delicious, to feed my hungry horde, I decided to give Mum a call. She had a recipe repertoire to rival the great chefs of Europe; every delectable dinner from *The Margaret Fulton Cookbook* was tried and tested by my mother and etched into her psyche. Mum was a veritable guru of home cookery, knowing the art of how to whip up something from nothing in no time and present it on matching plates ready for her hungry family to enjoy.

I loved these early evening chats with Mum. I hadn't spoken to her for a couple of days, so we'd have lots to talk about. I poured myself a cup of tea, grabbed a snack, got comfortable and dialled her number.

'Hello?'

'Hi!'

'Who's that?'

'Hi, Mum, it's me!'

'Who?'

'Sarah.'

'Oh, hi, darling.'

She seemed vague and didn't sound herself at all. I asked about her day and she couldn't recall what she'd been up to. It was her daily custom to 'pop up to the shops' so I asked her if she'd seen anyone she knew there, thinking it might jog her memory. No, she didn't remember going shopping or, as a matter of fact, doing anything at all that day. This was strange.

I steered the conversation to food and asked what she and Dad were having for dinner – something Mum loved to talk about. She didn't know.

Mum seemed uncomfortable chatting and clearly was in no mood for small talk. This was so unlike her. I probed her for answers and enquired about how she was feeling. Brushing it off and assuring me she was fine, she then uttered the strangest words of the evening: 'Sarah, darling, I'm just going to pop Dad on the phone. Love you lots, bye.'

'What? Dad? Why? But Mum, I rang to talk to …'

I was ready for one of our usual lengthy gabs. It wasn't that I didn't like talking to Dad. It was just that he and I preferred face-to-face catchups. Mum would give him all the news and keep him up to date. If I called and Dad answered, he'd say a quick hi and then hand the receiver straight to Mum. That was just what always happened.

Dad seemed as confused as I was, being thrust onto the telephone, thinking I had something of great importance to impart.

'No, I'd just rung to say hi.'

We were both a little bewildered at this turn of events but decided not to make a big deal of it, chalking it up to a one-off, before saying our goodbyes.

THE REAL JEANNIE SOMERVILLE

As a toddler, my precious daughter used to say to me, 'Mum, if I could walk into a shop and choose any other mum in the whole wide world, I'd still choose you.'

That's exactly how I feel about my mother.

My mum, Jeannie Margaret Somerville (nee O'Dea), is the best mum in the 'wold', as I wrote to her one Mother's Day and continued to write in her cards since then. I always thought she should write a textbook on parenting because I think – and I'm sure my brother Ben would agree – she did a cracker of a job bringing us up. Not to diminish the role our dad, Tony, had in our rearing, because he also played an important part and did a brilliant job. It would be fair to say, though, that Mum did shoulder the main task of raising the kids.

For Mum, every day was an opportunity to learn. Not only did she love learning herself, but she was passionate about instilling that love of grasping something previously unknown – the thrill of understanding a new concept for the very first time – in us, her kids. The world was her classroom and ours. Explaining something over our breakfast-time bacon and eggs, her face would light up when the penny dropped for us. 'Isn't that fascinating?' she would gush. There was always a pen and pad close at hand so Mum could draw an explanatory diagram to add further meaning and bring some new concept to life for us. I vividly remember sitting at the kitchen table and chatting with Mum long after we'd digested the last of our dinner, including our ice cream (with chocolate sauce, crushed nuts, hundreds and thousands and a sprinkle of Milo for good measure, which we were NEVER allowed to mash or stir. That's one thing I never understood and now, as an adult, feel almost compelled to do, just because I can – sorry, Mum!).

Lots of parents dread having the old 'birds and bees' conversation with their kids, putting it off until necessity knocks and their already pimply teenagers are hearing more than they need to know in the school playground. By the time their parents awkwardly open a copy of *What's Happening to Me?* they are already painfully aware of what's happening to them. Not so for Mum. As far as she was concerned, kids should be taught about ALL their body parts, regardless of whether they were classified as private or otherwise.

'You teach your kids about their arms and legs and what *they* do,' she would declare, 'so why leave out a whole section of their body and what *it* does?'

Good point. She taught us about what everything did. It was matter of fact; medical, even. Nothing gross or icky. By the time I was in primary school I had a detailed knowledge of vas deferens, fallopian tubes, ovaries and all things reproductive. My nanna once complimented five-year-old me on a beautiful picture of a pear that I'd drawn. She nearly fell off her chair when I thanked her but politely pointed out it was 'actually a uterus, Nanna, not a pear'.

Mum loved to point things out to us along the way as well. 'Look at those exquisite hydrangeas!' or 'There's a platypus – did you know that's one of only two mammals that lays eggs?' She'd give us maths problems as we were folding the washing: 'How many times can you fold that hanky symmetrically?'; or on a long drive up the coast: 'If we're going at 80 kilometres an hour and we have 200 kilometres until we reach our destination, how long will it take us to get there?' There was always something to learn – no matter how trivial – where Mum was concerned.

Speaking of trivia, Mum was a trivia champion. It was our life-long ambition to secretly enter Mum on *Sale of the Century*. Ben and I had visions of being driven around our local neighbourhood in our newly acquired Merc, which Mum would have won, and I always longed to turn up to school sporting a 'diamond-studded memento' pinned to my uniform.

Every night without fail, from 7 pm sharp, Mum, along with the rest of our family, would be glued to the box, eagerly awaiting Tony Barber's energetic, air-punching romp onto the set of our favourite show. It was a ritual and one that Mum was never happy about missing. Remember, back in the dark days before video recorders, you only had one shot at hearing each question, so silence was a prerequisite when the quiz show was in full swing. *'Ssshhh!'*

Now, perhaps my memory has embellished this over the years, but I seem to remember Mum getting every question right. There was scarcely anything trivial that was outside her realm of knowledge. She was truly amazing! It was in the 'Fame Game' that she really excelled. Sometimes she'd have an early stab at it when Tony Barber would excitedly pose the question, 'Who Am I?' Amid hand-waving to quieten Ben and me down, rolling her eyes when we shouted, 'Tony Barber!', Mum would already know the answer by the time he said, 'I was born in Mildura in 1933 ...' Long after Mum had confidently blasted it out, the contestant would finally echo her correct response and get a pick of the famous faces. Despite her obvious talent for tricky trivia, however, Mum refused to apply to go on the show and said she didn't know what she'd do to us if we ever thought about doing it for her! Our diamond-studded-memento-filled-dreams, up in smoke.

* * *

One of the major things Mum and Dad taught us was the utter necessity of a sense of humour. Dad would kill me if I didn't mention here his encyclopaedic knowledge of jokes and the fact that, given any topic, he can whip out a relevant gag (or two!) in under a minute flat. He's a true master of the story-telling joke, as anyone who knows him will attest. Mum's specialty, though, was The Pun. She was, in fact, the Queen of The Pun. Mum could pun with the best of them and would still be throwing up quality offerings long after everyone else had run dry. Ben and I were constantly being thrown into a pun-off and had to think on our feet, lest the Queen take us down. Mum could make a joke in, and of, any situation and was constantly cracking us up. She had a lightning-fast wit. I always admired Mum's ability to make me (and everyone around her) laugh. She could've been a stand-up comedian.

* * *

From an early age, Mum would tell me how very much she loved me, not only on a daily basis, but sometimes on the hour, every hour. There was never a skerrick of doubt in my mind that Mum loved me (and Ben) with her whole, overflowing, unconditional and fiercely loyal heart. If ever there was a question over our suitability for a task, even if we doubted our own ability for the job at hand, Mum would loudly proclaim our credentials and insist that we could do anything we put our minds to. She was a self-esteem builder of inordinate proportions. Continually hearing that we were 'gorgeous', 'beautiful', 'clever', 'funny', 'capable' and 'talented', among countless other adulations, built in us a certain confidence and resilience that I'm grateful for to this day.

Although her constant praise was biased and some might say over the top, she made us believe we were worthy of her love, giving us total security in who we were. I can't speak for Ben here, but it gave me the sense that I didn't ever have to prove myself to anyone. I was loved unconditionally and totally just the way I was. No matter what happened, we knew Mum would always remain our biggest fan. That's such an incredible gift!

Along these lines, Mum taught us it was always better to be a leader than a follower and in this she led by example. She implored us not to be sheep and encouraged us to have the courage of our convictions. Even if we were alone in those convictions and the hum of the madding crowd was suggesting a plan of action to the contrary, Mum wanted us to be sure of what we believed and to stick to it with confidence. Standing boldly and resolutely in the face of peer group pressure was never a big deal for me. I am grateful to Mum for equipping me in this way.

Mum's fierce loyalty and abundant love were also poured out upon her wider family. She adored her three siblings Patty, John and Donny, and was equally enamoured with her nieces and nephews, forming a particular bond with Patty's girls, Andrea and Meredith, with whom we spent a lot of time when we were growing up. Both Mum and Dad embraced as part of the family my husband, Ross, and Ben's wife, Julie, from the minute they came on the scene, always showing them love and support. As breeders, Ben and I certainly did our bit (so to speak) in increasing the Family

Dynasty. With our partners we produced seven grandchildren for Mum and Dad. Our son Sam was the first grandchild on the scene, his adoring grandparents enduring hours in the hospital waiting room eagerly (read: impatiently) awaiting his much-anticipated arrival. Our daughter Molly, equally adored, was born two years later, followed by Toby, our gorgeous third child (potentially named 'Tarzan' had his doting siblings had their way), who was born three years later in the year 2000. Just as we had given away our pram and found good homes for all our various baby paraphernalia our precious little Maisy brought us great joy by gracing us with her presence six years later, to complete our bonny, bouncing brood.

By the time Cathy Freeman and Ian Thorpe had streaked to gold-medal stardom at the Sydney Olympics, Ben and Julie had welcomed their beautiful first-born, Sophie into the world. Sophie was blessed with her little cherub cheeked sister, Emily a couple of years later, followed by their new playmate and darling brother Will, born just four months before our Maisy. I'm delighted to say that all seven cousins (along with Sophie's husband Tom and daughter Rachel) are all super close friends and enjoy one another's company regularly.

Mum relished time spent with her grandchildren, involving herself completely in their lives, just as she had with us. Until each of my four children were school-aged, Mum looked after them on Fridays – a day they always looked forward to. She and Dad came to Presentation Days, sat through ballet concerts and cheered loudly and enthusiastically from the sporting sidelines, always beaming with pride over what their grandchildren were achieving.

Another of Mum's great qualities was her ability to have fun. Walking hand-in-hand with her raucous sense of humour was her natural tendency towards being the life of the party. It would always be fun if Mum was there. She could turn every occasion into something memorable. At my twenty-first birthday party she taught a crowded dance floor how to do 'The Pony', frolicking around, hooves aloft, stopping every now and then to toss her imaginary mane. It was hilarious! She was always a woman of very few inhibitions. Video footage from our wedding has Mum arm-in-arm with a couple of our friends, belting out an AC/DC classic at high voltage, complete with the requisite head-banging moves.

While her inhibitions may have been few, her integrity was high. Mum was something of a morals warrior, ensuring that Ben and I were well-versed in right and wrong. She drummed into us the importance of being trustworthy, honest, hard-working and true to your word.

It was my secret fantasy to one day perform a citizen's arrest and I'm sure that desire came from watching my mum in action. I vividly recall witnessing some young criminals-in-the-making stuffing their jumpers with enough packs of coveted Rugby League footy cards to fill a suitcase. Mum gave them the evil eye and while their consciences were obviously pricked, they continued to stuff the said cards up their fronts until they were so padded out, they wouldn't have been out of place in a *Biggest Loser* line-up. I watched in awe as Mum glided towards them and with a loud 'What do you think you're doing?' had those boys so rattled they coughed up all the cards and drew the attention of the supermarket staff, who had them frisked within an inch of their lives. Justice prevailed. I like to think Mum might've been responsible for setting the boys on the right path and averting them from the life of crime they'd have been destined to lead had they not been stopped in their tracks by Jeannie Somerville.

Mum's older, adored sister, my Auntie Patty, was a bit of a Light-Finger Lucy herself, much to Mum's dismay. She travelled a lot, staying at posh hotels, and would often boast about her latest acquisitions when we went to visit. She was thrilled to have nearly collected an entire set of scotch glasses, obtained over the years through holidaying repeatedly at the same hotel. Patty also had quite a collection of bathrobes and beach towels from various tropical locations. Mum was fighting a losing battle trying to turn her wayward sister around. Patty thought it was hilarious; I was horrified (but that's understandable, given whose daughter I was).

It irritated Mum no end when people took it upon themselves to open packets and sample things in the supermarket. 'That's stealing!' she would proclaim loudly through the crowded aisles, her words creating an echo that bounced off the fun-size Mars Bars and resounded all the way back to the Space Food Sticks.

We would often encounter mothers who were dreaded 'packet-openers', handing their children treats to console them through their harrowing grocery shopping ordeals. 'I hope you intend to pay for that!' Mum would say.

If Mum had any inkling they may have been trying to get away with not paying – by hiding the packets in their pockets, for instance – it wouldn't be uncommon for her to wheel the old trolley around, Ben and I in tow, feeling like we were part of a real-life cop show, and give chase. Keeping our trolley at a safe distance so as not to arouse suspicion, all the while fixing a watchful eye on the culprit, she would close in at the checkout. When the pocketed packet was inevitably 'overlooked', Mum would give them a timely reminder that they might also like to pay for the already consumed, concealed item that just happened to be in their pocket. Though some kids may (understandably) have found this mortifying, I filled with pride, humming a hybrid of the Meadow Lea and Tip Top bread ads to myself as we strolled down the aisles in the knowledge that we were a crack team, bringing justice to the suburbs. Good on, Mum. She really did need to be congratulated.

* * *

To say Mum loved words would be an understatement of grand proportions. She was a wordsmith, an avid reader (as was Dad) and her vocabulary was bigger than the Pacific Ocean. Words were a ubiquitous part of our growing up. Dad delighted in coming to the dinner table armed with the latest gargantuan words he'd found in his recent reading material, his linguistic gymnastics delighting everyone (no one more so than himself). He'd be (not so) secretly swotting up, hoping to have unearthed a single unit of language that was not yet in Mum's repertoire. He rarely succeeded but was oh-so chuffed when he did. Mum would then bone up on its Latin roots and derivations and proceed to use it in any relevant sentence she could for the next month, at least, as would Dad.

Ben and I loved to play the Dictionary Game with Mum. We'd open the trusty *Oxford Dictionary* at a random page and see if we could stump the old girl with a word she'd never heard before. She was amazing! From medical terms and bizarre phobias to geological definitions and rare African bird names – you name it, Mum knew them all. Well, almost all. There was barely a noun, verb or adjective beyond her comprehension.

Another of Mum's favourite games to play with us was the Word Association Game. We'd each take turns to say a word and then it was the job of the next person to say the very first word that came into their head, thus revealing their hidden associations. She would delight in psychoanalysing us afterwards – as we debriefed, she would try to get to the bottom of why we associated one particular thing with another. Somehow, we'd always end up associating something with the toilet. I wonder what that says about us.

Charades was also a Somerville family favourite, driven by Mum, of course. On Friday afternoons, more often than not, Ben and I would be delighted to arrive home from school to find a note in Mum's copperplate-neat, loopy handwriting, instructing us to 'Come round to Jill's place.' We'd make our way to the home of our good family friends, the Livingstones, knowing we'd be in for a fun night. Their neighbours, the Smiths, would also come over and we'd grab some Chinese takeaway and play charades well into the night. We had lots of laughs.

There was a famous night when one of us held up six fingers, having only just revealed, through the classic mime where one hand curls around an eye to make an eyepiece while the other fist winds an imaginary crank around the opposite ear, that the phrase was a movie title. Without a further sound or syllable being mimed, someone yelled out *'One Flew Over the Cuckoo's Nest'* – which was indeed the correct answer! This had us rolling around on the floor, laughing uncontrollably. Forevermore, whenever we got together and someone had trouble coming up with something to mime, one of us only had to hold up the six fingers and peals of laughter would ensue as together we chorused the title of the Jack Nicholson favourite.

To say that Mum's love affair with words also made her partial to the odd crossword was certainly an understatement. She completed them in their entirety, effortlessly and regularly. If the daily crossword in the paper hadn't sated her appetite, she'd invest in a *Woman's Day* or *New Idea* to quench her crossword passion. Once she cottoned on to *Bumper Puzzle* books at the newsagent's, she was on cloud nine! Filling in 'acrosses and downs' and deciphering cryptic clues was what Mum loved to do best of all in her down time. Sadly for her, and not for lack of trying, Mum was never able to pass on to her offspring the art of the enigma that is the cryptic crossword. She would spend hours pointing out hidden anagrams, double meanings and clever twists to me but, for the life of me, I just couldn't get it. Sorry, Mum.

Still on the theme of words, poetry was another one of Mum's passions and skills. She loved the rhythm of a well-written poem. She'd always be getting us to compose limericks around the kitchen table and was a very good poet herself (though she didn't know it). One of my all-time favourites of Mum's limericks was:

There was a young woman begat
Three babies named Nat, Pat and Tat.
It was fun in the breeding,
But hell in the feeding,
When she found there was no tit for Tat!

Mum had a whole swag of cute little ditties, sayings and songs that she imparted to us, intentionally or otherwise, over the years. It never ceased to amaze me how many of these one brain could contain. While she was peeling potatoes or expertly crumbing the chicken at the kitchen bench, silly song after silly song would flow forth from her mouth, interspersed with show tunes and songs from her favourite movies. It isn't surprising that I find myself now, in my middle age, belting out these tunes and humming along to many of Mum's little ditties as I peel my own potatoes. I hope my kids will one day do the same.

Another of Mum's admirable traits was her ability to keep lots of proverbial balls in the air at one time. To keep the ball analogy going, she was always on the ball and never dropped the ball. Now that I think of it, she could've been a juggling rugby player. She missed her calling. Mum handled all the complexities of raising a busy family, looking after our needs before we even asked her. She mastered the logistics of knowing where we had to be and what was on, and would get us there on time. She always knew where we were and who we were with and was across everyone's ever-changing schedules.

She cooked us gourmet meals every night, chauffeured us around to every one of our extra-curricular comings and goings, paid the bills, kept the house spotless, volunteered on the school canteen (how good were the free lunches?) and was an active member of the school P&C. Mum helped us with all our homework, taking a real interest in what we were learning. She would read the books we were reading at school, discuss with us the history we were studying, and practice the maths formulas we were swatting. She was eternally involved and interested.

As Ben and I grew older and began venturing out after dark, Mum usually tried to stay up for us, even if we were due home late. On the odd occasion when her stamina waned and she could no longer keep those droopy eyelids peeled, Ben and I would always be met with a very cute note, written in Mum's impeccable handwriting – usually on paper towel – saying, 'Please wake me when you come home.' As the years went on this would become 'P.W.M.W.Y.C.H.'

We would dutifully creep into her room and give her a reassuring nudge to alert her of our safe homecoming, at which she would proceed to ask us some rapid-fire questions about our night: who had been there, had we had fun, what was everyone wearing, what did you have to eat, was there any dancing ...? It would always culminate with a yawning Mum uttering, 'That's lovely, darling ...' and then she'd drift back off to sound slumber. The amazing thing was, the next day Mum would always remember what we'd told her in the wee hours. She showed a genuine interest in our friends. She loved it when we had the hoards over and always encouraged it,* mingling and chatting with everyone, eliciting a few laughs along the way. Our friends all got along with Mum. She was a pretty likeable character, after all.

---

*Well, there was that one time, though ... I had a slumber party with about ten friends and we spilt a can of Coke on the brand-new white shag pile. That was after explicit instructions from Mum that: 'There was to be no eating or drinking in the lounge room!' The entire can of carpet shampoo we sprayed enthusiastically on the spreading brown patch, which despite giving off a fresh Spring fragrance, didn't go a long way towards rectifying the unsightly blemish. We had a strategically placed pot plant over the stain forevermore. Pity it was in the middle of the room. Oops. Sorry, Mum.

If there was ever an award ceremony for tact, my mother would have been a hot contender. Measured and compassionate when she dealt with others' feelings, Mum had the skill of being honest in a caring and sensitive way. She taught us to walk in the shoes of others (not literally, of course, unless the shoes were gorgeous and they were offering); she would always encourage us to imagine how they'd have felt. If someone was struggling with their weight, Mum would empathise and understand how tough it could be to lose excess kilos once they'd crept on. If someone was behaving rudely, she would ponder what might have happened in their life to cause them to behave that way. If someone was going through a hardship of any kind and Mum heard about it, she could barely stop herself from shedding a loving tear for them. She was such a compassionate soul.

STRANGE HAPPENINGS

After Mum and Dad retired, they enjoyed a busy social life, often going to the movies and eating out, spending time with their grandkids and each other. They were so regular at the local yum cha restaurant, they'd be welcomed with open arms by their favourite waiter, with whom they were on a first-name basis. Then they'd be escorted promptly to their usual table.

They had a lovely trip to Europe, travelled to New Zealand with their good friends and took a cruise off the Caribbean. They holidayed at regular intervals in their beloved holiday unit in Surfers Paradise, meeting up with their Queensland buddies each night for a drink at their local watering hole, the D'Arcy Arms. They enjoyed all the fun and exciting things you'd expect after spending a good part of their lives working hard and raising a family. There would be no lounging around watching daytime telly. Mum and Dad saw their long-awaited escape from work as a time to kick back and enjoy their new-found leisure time and freedom.

It was around this time that we noticed a few odd things happening. Without a doubt, Mum's hearing started to dwindle. She was constantly saying, 'Eh?', and if she had her back to you, you may as well have been conversing with a tree. Dad took her to a hearing specialist to see if her aural faculties were up to scratch and check if it was all in our imaginations. Well, the results came back as a resounding gong (though Mum didn't hear it): Mum only had 30 per cent of her hearing! Thirty per cent. Not 30 per cent gone, but only 30 per cent left. That's pretty low by anyone's standards. No wonder her favourite word was, 'Eh?'

Uncharacteristically, and despite the doctor's definitive evidence to the contrary, Mum refused to believe there was anything wrong with her hearing. This seemed ridiculous to all of us. Any mention of, dare I say it ... a hearing aid, was like a dirty word to Mum and she wouldn't have a bar of it. We tried to use reason: 'You already wear glasses to help with reading, Mum.' But when we said, 'A hearing aid will just be like glasses, only for your ears ...' all Mum heard was '*Blah, blah, blah* ...' and her response was an emphatic, 'No. No. No.'

* * *

Talking on the telephone is so old school these days but it was our mum's favourite mode of communication. The next best thing to chatting face-to-face was nattering on the phone for hours. At least twice a week, I'd pick up the receiver to hear Mum's soothing, familiar voice, and we'd exchange our latest news and solve the problems of the world. If I needed advice, she was my first port of call. Did she think I'd been too hard on one of the kids? How should I respond in a certain situation? Should I wear the blue dress or the yellow one to the party on Saturday night? What else, apart from flour, did you put in a white sauce again? I looked forward to our chats.

With Mum's capacity for listening slowly ebbing away, conversing over the phone was becoming more and more of a challenge. I could sense that she was just responding by rote at some points in the conversation, with well-placed 'Ohs' and 'I sees' sprinkled in at appropriate intervals. The fact that she couldn't hear us entirely was made abundantly clear when she was in the midst of a long call with our daughter, Molly. After responding to Mum's 'How are you, darling?' with 'Oh, I've had a pretty bad day, Nanna, and I'm not feeling too well', Mum enthusiastically replied, 'Oh, that's lovely, darling!' Huh?

Our phone calls became briefer, to the point where, as I have mentioned, Mum would hand the phone to Dad! Instead of the usual hasty greeting from Dad, followed by a quick catch-up and a prompt handover to Mum for the duration of the call, suddenly the reverse was taking place. Mum was answering the call and before I'd have a chance to say 'Jack Robinson', she'd announce, 'I'll put you on to your father.' Dad became a kind of interpreter, which was very strange for both of us. Not that I don't like chatting to Dad, of course, but this was the first of many bizarre role reversals.

Mum had always taken responsibility for the finances in our house – paying the bills, reconciling the cheque books, keeping tabs on the accounts. Dad deferred to her and sought her opinion on all matters financial. For as long as I could remember, it was Mum who'd had her finger on the proverbial pulse. Jim, an old family friend, would make an annual visit to our humble abode and, in exchange for a couple of ice-cold cans, would help out with lodging the family's tax returns, super fund management and that sort of thing. This had been happening for twenty years. Jim began to notice, after decades of Mum being the more enthusiastic recipient of his financial advice, that she had started to take a back seat, deferring to Dad and seeming less interested in financial matters. He told me that, previously, while Dad was always present at their meetings, Mum had actively managed all aspects of the super fund. She maintained the records and dealt with any day-to-day decisions relating to their accounts and finances.

On the last occasion Jim and my parents met together, he told me that Mum had 'completely withdrawn her involvement and refused to provide any input, deferring all decisions to Tony', my dad. This was the complete opposite to the way they'd always operated. Over a two-year period, Jim observed a rapid decline in both her 'presentation and mental capacity', he said. That was an interesting and perceptive observation from someone who only saw Mum and Dad once a year.

Dad also remarked that he had seen a gradual withdrawal in Mum, noticing a general decline in her awareness and understanding of the family's financial matters.

WHAT'S GOING ON?

I now know, through researching Mum's condition, that craving sweet or fatty foods, and bingeing on them, or on alcohol or cigarettes, are typical symptoms to expect from someone suffering from dementia. For my mother it was alcohol. Though my parents had always been drinkers, it's fair to say they typically drank in moderation. Mum would often sip a glass of wine while she was cooking dinner and perhaps top up her glass over a meal and Dad would have a couple of beers – ice-cold libations, as he called them – when he got home from work. During this period of strange happenings, however, Mum was frequently indulging in a little too much wine. She would often ring us late in the evening, slurring her words and barely able to string a sentence together.

This was alarming, as we had no diagnosis to link her strange behaviour to at the time. What was happening? Was our mother becoming an alcoholic?

Dad would dutifully report to us, revealing the excessive

amounts of alcohol Mum was consuming – sometimes a bottle of wine a night – but found himself seemingly unable to convince her to do otherwise. Ben and I urged him to stop Mum from buying alcohol, but he struggled with taking what he saw as a 'pleasure' away from her. He was even buying bottles of wine to appease her. Mum's drinking was becoming more of an issue as time marched on; Dad's distress grew, but he remained unwilling to take action.

When Mum clocked up seventy rotations around the sun, Ben and I decided it was cause for a special celebration and made plans to indulge her on a weekend getaway to Melbourne, with just the two of us. You don't turn seventy every day. I must admit, I was a tad nervous about the whole drinking issue, but thought we'd just play it by ear.

Being a regular jetsetter for work, Ben had visited Melbourne more times than you could poke a blunt stick at and had put together a jam-packed itinerary for the three of us Sydneysiders, allowing us to fully acquaint ourselves with this hip and happening southern metropolis. Our accommodation was an excellent launching pad for our sight-seeing expeditions, primarily on foot. We chatted as we meandered along the banks of the Yarra. We shook with laughter at Dame Edna in concert. We engaged in civilised conversation over high tea at the Windsor and punned while prancing through parklands. We reminisced about times gone by while indulging in fine food and generally had an absolute ball. It was just like old times.

Mum had a glass of wine with dinner but our fears of her having a 'drinking problem' were allayed, as she seemed completely satisfied not to indulge further. Looking back now, this was probably the last time we got to spend quality time with Mum as her true self; memories we will forever cherish and play over in our minds. For those two days, Mum was back in all her glory.

* * *

Dad (along with Ben and I) had the ongoing pleasure, for many years, of being a daily recipient of Mum's fabulous cooked breakfasts, among numerous other gourmet meals she'd whip up for him. His fast was broken each morning with a mouth-watering array of bacon, eggs, sausages, cutlets, tomatoes, toast ... It was a mixed-grill feast fit for a king. One morning around this time, Dad descended the stairs, his nostrils assaulted with the delicious aromas he'd become accustomed to. He and Mum enjoyed their morning morsels together, then packed away the kitchen, ready to get on with the day.

Shortly afterwards, you can imagine Dad's surprise when he once again had his senses accosted by the sound and smell of sizzling bacon – an encore performance he neither expected nor could explain. He gently enquired as to why Mum was cooking breakfast again, but his enquiry was met with an emphatic, if not a little aggressive, 'What are you talking about, Tony?' She denied having cooked breakfast only a short time before and honestly believed this was the first time that day she'd flipped an egg or skewered a snag. Dad realised that arguing was pointless, but argued nonetheless.

He rang us shortly after, to recount what had happened, and we too were confused. What was going on?

Chinese food was a regular Saturday night indulgence for our family while Ben and I were growing up. The Glenrose Chinese – our local felt-wallpapered restaurant, complete with bow-tied waiters (we had a soft spot for Colin), red napkins and big round tables – cooked our favourite fare. We'd partake in ham and chicken rolls, prawn cutlets, Mongolian lamb and boneless lemon chicken on a regular basis. The serving of San Choy Bow always made us giggle, though Ben may not agree. When Colin the waiter would turn up at our table with his nest of neatly trimmed lettuce leaf receptacles, he would distribute them the same way each time, the sizes corresponding directly with our ages. As he carefully tonged the leaves one by one into our bowls, the ritual would start with Dad's oversized foliage – barely containable in the little bowl – and would culminate, as a barely visible leaf was placed in Ben's bowl, with Colin's announcement: 'Small leaf for the small boy.' We could almost recite the menu word for word. Ben would often declare himself to be completely full, though when Dad would predictably say, 'Oh, well I guess that means you won't want dessert?' Ben would convince us that he had a separate 'dessert compartment' in his stomach, not affected in the least by the over-indulgences he'd heaped into his little bowl. He always finished the night with a crescendo of deep-fried ice cream. We knew this restaurant well, to say the least.

It is for this reason that Dad was perplexed when Mum volunteered to go and pick up the takeaway one night, only to return home after around half an hour, bewildered and totally empty handed, declaring she had forgotten where the Chinese restaurant was. This was weird. Very weird.

One night, Mum, Dad and I attended a gig in Manly where Ben's newly formed rock band was playing. He had struck up friendships with some fellow dads at his children's school and they had discovered on a family camping trip that they could combine their mutual love of music and complementary talents to sound 'not too shabby at all'. Mum and Dad couldn't have been prouder as their handsome son strode on to the stage and began crooning sweetly while strumming his six-string. My sister-in-law's parents were there too.

No sooner had they started playing than Mum began to swear at the top of her voice. 'How ¥@$&%# good are they? You @$?&#% rock!' You get the picture. Chopper Read would've been blushing. For some, this behaviour might be totally normal, but our mother hated swearing. She despised it. She never swore. This was bizarre. Everyone who knew her was shocked (and possibly mildly amused at the incongruity of it all).

Strange things like these kept happening. Mum would walk to

the shops and then spend an hour in the carpark trying to locate her car, which was tucked up safely at home, a few kilometres away, in the garage. Or vice versa; she would drive to the shops and then walk home, the fact that she had taken the car completely slipping her mind.

Once, she parked outside her friend Jill's house and from there walked to do her grocery shopping. When she couldn't find her car in the carpark, Mum placed a distress call to Dad, who immediately came to pick her up, suspecting they'd fallen victim to a gang of car-jacking hooligans. Scoping the area for the said hooligans, Dad inadvertently spied Mum's car, sitting pretty, right outside Jill's house. Actually, Jill's old house. In fact, Jill hadn't lived there for over ten years. Mum could in no way explain her actions. She seemed just as perplexed as her poor husband.

THE D-WORD

As Dad reported these instances to us in due time, I must admit, the D-word began to float around in my consciousness. I think this was the case for most of us, though no one could verbalise it. Mum's drinking continued to be heavy, particularly so when out with friends. On more than one occasion, she completely ironed herself out and had to be carried back to the car. Dad is a weightlifter and has been since he was nineteen – to ward off the bullies that kicked sand in his face at the beach, as legend would have it. But even so, he had to enlist the help of some equally burly blokes to assist him in getting his wife back to the car when she was particularly inebriated. Mum also suffered some nasty falls after imbibing a little too much vino, including one particularly bad tumble down a flight of concrete stairs. She was battered and bruised and had to bandage her sprained wrist. Yet, when we enquired about what had happened, she said she wasn't sure.

We began to notice other subtle behavioural changes – Mum

became noticeably more aggressive, her fuse much shorter than usual. At first, we assumed this was due to the drinking (which certainly exacerbated it), but it became increasingly worse. Rightly or wrongly, some friends began to withdraw, perhaps out of fear or a lack of understanding of how to deal with the situation and clearly sensing that change was afoot. Mum was a little hard to be around now. She became quite withdrawn and her love of crosswords became nothing short of an obsession. I now know that this behaviour is common for those suffering from frontal lobe dementia.

It's a widely known fact that the worst possible question you can ask a woman who is carrying a little extra padding is, 'When is the baby due?' I ought to know; I've found out the hard way, beaming with excitement and proclaiming my delight at the fantastic prospect of a new family member, only to be told in a deflated tone, 'No, I'm still fat from my last baby.' Oh, the shame! Well, the worst possible question we could ask Mum at this time was: 'Is there anything wrong?' She vehemently denied the possibility that any conceivable thing could be amiss. The more we tried to reason, the louder she'd protest. The more we tried to point out her uncharacteristic behaviours, the more adamant and cantankerous she became. We knew she desperately needed to see a doctor, but she refused to go. She insisted she was fine.

A couple of more alarming things happened to further cement in our minds that we really needed to get Mum to the doctor. One sunny afternoon, she decided it would be a good idea to cook a little mixed grill. She piled the kitchen hotplate with succulent sausages, plump chops and juicy lamb cutlets and cranked the dial to high. She then proceeded to lock every door and window in the house and go upstairs to her bedroom for the night. The fact that it was broad daylight aside, the mixed grill was sizzling away unsupervised while Dad lazed by the pool reading his novel, totally oblivious to the goings on inside the house. Oblivious, that is, until he was jolted out of relaxation mode by the ear-piercing smoke alarms whistling at a high decibel from the kitchen. Unable to enter through the locked back door, he tried windows and other doors – but to no avail. Mum had achieved a Fort Knox-worthy lock-up, and no one was breaking into that joint.

By now, black smoke was visible in the house and Dad could smell burning meat. It had cycled through medium-rare, medium-well, well-done … and was on its way to being able to be carbon dated, way beyond resembling anything remotely edible. Dad called the fire brigade, who rushed to his aid, jimmying open a window and saving the house and his wife, who was soundly slumbering despite the smoke alarms blasting from every room in the house, sounding out through the surrounding suburbs. Now, that's what I call 'out like a light'. The fire fighters told Dad it was a narrow escape.

Then Dad began noticing small dings on Mum's car, which she explained away, suggesting the negligence belonged to someone wielding a wonky trolley in the carpark or to another careless driver. He didn't buy it. One day she slammed into a gutter and lost the hub cap off one of the wheels. Rather than telling Dad straight away, Mum went ahead and let her fingers do the walking, ringing someone she found in the *Yellow Pages* to arrange a replacement wheel. Now, ordinarily this would have been a commendable idea; though in this instance, unfortunately, Mum didn't write down the name of the wheel-dealer, or any details whatsoever about the repair. Consequently, when Dad received a message on his answering machine from a mysterious tyre seller, telling him his tyre was ready to collect and could he please pick it up, he had no idea what had been repaired, where it was or what to do. There was no phone number, no name, no idea. Suffice to say, they never did get that wheel fixed.

* * *

Halitosis is fairly common among people of Mum's age and nothing a quick mint or brush of the teeth can't eradicate, at least temporarily. I began to notice, however, that Mum's breath had taken a turn for the worse. My suggestions of 'Here, Mum, have a mint' were embraced, but no mint would come anywhere near fixing this issue. I'd liken it to popping a couple of tissues down to soak up the oil spewing from the reef-stricken *Exxon Valdez*. There had also been some recent mutterings from Dad regarding Mum's reluctance to shower, and I had noticed a slight odour clinging to her clothes and hair. This was an awkward topic to broach; no one wants to point out to their own mother that she may have some personal hygiene issues.

Over the previous year or so, Mum had been shedding kilos at a rapid rate. At first she insisted it was simply 'portion control', as they say in the weight-loss business, but she was becoming alarmingly thin. We quizzed Dad as to whether Mum was in fact consuming normal meals. Unfortunately, he hadn't noticed. Mum would bring his dinner to him while he was watching TV and then slip away to watch her program in the other room, where Dad assumed she was also munching down on some evening sustenance. It seemed she wasn't. Whether this was a result of forgetfulness or an effort to stay thin, we're not sure. She did comment that she didn't have a huge appetite.

We were watching an episode of *The Biggest Loser* together one night, witnessing the contestants working themselves into the ground in an effort to return their bodies and lives to some semblance of normality. Mum announced, most uncharacteristically, that these 'fat people' were 'disgusting'. I was incredulous at what had just come out of Mum's mouth and tried to explain the beauty of the show in helping people out of their ruts, exposing the real reasons obesity had them in its clutches. Mum refused to listen and kept insisting they only had themselves to blame for being 'fat'.

I was shocked. This was so unlike my mother. It left me

questioning all I'd known of my mum. Had she turned away from the values she had worked so hard to instil in me and that I now clung to? But how could one's core values be so fluid? I found myself grappling with the evolution that was taking place. Desperate for some clarity, a medical opinion now seemed crucial.

THE DIAGNOSIS

Eventually, after much cajoling, Dad managed to convince Mum to see her local doctor. I'm still not sure how he did it. The doctor ordered scans of various kinds and referred Mum to a specialist, whose specialty I must confess I'd never heard of: he was a geriatrician, a doctor for geriatrics – obvious once you know. It was strange to think of my mum as a geriatric. In my head, she was still in her forties and I was in my twenties! The first appointment with Dr Gerry didn't exactly go swimmingly. Mum and Dad went together to see the good doctor and all our secret fears were met with the diagnosis we'd been dreading.

Mum had dementia.

Oh, bugger.

Mum was outraged with this declaration that questioned her very sanity and she was suitably indignant. When Dr Gerry began to address the topic of Mum's overenthusiastic consumption of alcohol, things turned even more pear-shaped. Her indignation morphed into outrage. She stomped right out of the surgery, leaving Dr Gerry (and everyone else within a kilometre's radius) in no doubt about what she thought of his diagnosis and where exactly he could ... er, shove it.

Following this disastrous encounter, Dr Gerry requested a meeting with just Ben and me, to further discuss Mum's diagnosis in something of a less heated environment. We had next to no experience with dementia, each coming to this meeting with our own preconceived ideas about what it was. Consequently, we had high expectations for the clarity the doctor might impart.

Dr Gerry was friendly enough and showed us pictures of Mum's brain. It was quite confronting to see the sections of her brain that had already atrophied (literally, shrunk and wasted away as the cells had degenerated). He briefly explained that dementia was a broad umbrella term, under which many different dementia-related diseases lived. Mum's particular brand of dementia was frontotemporal dementia, also known as frontotemporal lobar degeneration (FTLD) or Pick's disease. As the name suggests, this form of dementia affects the frontal and temporal lobes of the brain. He briefly touched on the fact that this was the part of the brain that controlled mood, behaviour, organisation, judgement and self-control. Wow. Those seemed like fairly important, if not basic, functions that you wouldn't really want to live without.

Even though in our heart of hearts we'd known to expect this bad news, the physical evidence hit us like a ton of bricks. These were no happy snaps. This was our mother's glorious, clever, witty, intelligent brain withering away before our eyes and there was nothing we could do to stop the demon-march into her eventual decline. We were both close to tears.

We had a myriad of questions but didn't know where to start. We needed Dr Gerry to give us a handy page of Frequently Asked Questions, but instead he left us staring dumbfounded at one another, unsure of what to say. It reminded me of my first attempt at catching a train in the Paris Metro, with my repertoire of French words limited to *fête*, *café*, *croissant* and of course *répertoire*, an absence of a map of any kind and absolutely no clue where I was or where I was going. All I could do was gaze with glazed eyes at the list of foreign suburbs and place names and hope for the best.

We had barely scratched the surface when Dr Gerry abruptly changed the subject. Confusingly, he began talking about 'Guardianship' and 'Power of Attorney'. He was urging us to 'have things in order' for when Mum could no longer make her own decisions. This discussion felt way too premature. No sooner had we received the diagnosis than he was telling us Mum was about to die!

Of course, that wasn't really what he was saying, but that was certainly how I interpreted the gist of the conversation. I thought he was referring to Mum's will, which I was horrified he'd even bring up at such an emotional time. I was far more concerned with getting Mum some help and waiting for him to reveal some sort of miracle cure.

Our meeting with this doctor finished with an exhortation to get Mum to stop drinking. He told us her condition would worsen rapidly if she didn't stop and that if she could somehow curb her wild behaviour she'd have a much better chance of prolonging her days. He made it sound as if Mum had some sort of choice in the matter, her drinking akin to naughtiness that needed to be brought into line.

I know now it was a symptom of her dementia, caused by the diminishing self-control centre in her frontal lobes. He didn't tell us that. I've since had a lot of time to reflect on that meeting and the lack of advice and information we were given. We left his office with more fears than practical tips, more questions than answers. He told us nothing about symptoms or whether Mum should stay at home or go into care; he left us with no plan of action and no real understanding of what we were dealing with. Our homework was to stop Mum from drinking and to obtain Power of Attorney and Guardianship – whatever they were. End of meeting. All we knew was: Mum had dementia.

HEAD IN THE SAND

Ross and I and my brother Ben and his wife Julie became increasingly worried about Mum being left alone. Dad led quite an active social life, heading to the gym each morning, drinking at the pub with his mates in the afternoon, popping out here and there. He was often not at home. He insisted Mum would be fine alone. He also insisted she was more than able to keep cooking, even as she was becoming forgetful and leaving the hotplates on regularly. It was like saying, 'I'll just pop into the casino for a spot of roulette, maybe a few hands of poker; the kids will be just fine to wait in the car,' on a 40-degree day. It was anything but fine.

Despite our urgings, and even after the fire-brigade incident, Dad resisted our pleas and continued to leave Mum alone and ensconced in her role as head chef. She continued to wash and iron Dad's clothes, cook his meals and generally look after him and the house. In his defence, it must have been easier to remain in denial than to upset the apple cart after forty-nine years of matrimonial order and stability, not to mention very clearly defined roles.

But although Dad's attitude of complete denial was understandable, it was also a worry. When he had to fly up to Queensland for a little over a week and presumed Mum would be fine on her Pat Malone (with which Mum strongly concurred), Ross and I insisted that she come and stay with us. Neither of them was enamoured of this decision.

Well, to say that week was an eye-opener would be an understatement akin to saying the Great Wall of China is a nice little fence. The extent to which Dad had been downplaying Mum's condition became vastly and immediately apparent to us. Without a doubt, it was one of the toughest weeks of my life.

AN EYE-OPENER

It was a sunny morning when Dad dropped Mum at our place on his way to the airport, waving her off as he prepared to wing towards the tropical north. After taking Mum to her room, I offered to help unpack her bag and was caught between hysterical laughter and tears as I unzipped it to find an entire suitcase filled with shoes – a collection Imelda Marcos would no doubt have been proud of. There wasn't a shirt, skirt, pair of undies or toothbrush in sight. It was creative packing if nothing else. A quick trip back to the family home was in order, to fill in the missing gaps and fix the packing faux pas.

The entire time she was away from home, my mother insisted she did not need anyone to look after her. She was perfectly capable of being alone, thank you very much. She wanted to go home immediately and told us *ad nauseam*. Who were we to tell her what to do? She recalled the good old days when Dad, who spent the majority of his working life as a travelling salesman, would go away for three-week stretches, leaving her very capable self at home to keep the home fires burning. (In reality, she may have literally kept the home fires burning ... to the ground, if we'd left her there solo.) It was the most frustrating thing in the world, both for Mum, who sincerely saw no logic in being away from where she knew she belonged, and for us, trying to explain rationally that she wasn't able to look after herself anymore and couldn't be home alone. It just didn't make sense to her.

As the week ran its course, Mum became aggressively insistent that she be allowed to 'Go home!' She was looking dangerously thin by this time; wielding her massive suitcase (now stowing more than just her impressive shoe collection) out the door, threatening to 'Walk home if she bloody well had to', she was quite a sight to behold. Her luggage was almost as big as her! At one stage, she managed to lug it down the front stairs and was on her way back to where she lived. It was a 14-kilometre walk, mind you, which would have taken a good couple of hours even for the Hawaiian Iron Man Champion, let alone a woman in her seventies with a jumbo piece of luggage in tow.

We let her go for a few minutes and she made it across the road and down a few blocks before I sent my son to tail her on his skateboard and try to waylay her until we could bring the car around. That was the easy part. Mum's bloodcurdling screams certainly aroused the attention of the neighbours, as did her high-decibel pleas for someone to 'Stop this woman' (that was me, by the way) from 'kidnapping' or, even worse, 'abducting' her. I had her by the hand but didn't want to use force, especially with the whole suburb out among their front garden shrubbery, eyeing me with great suspicion, on the verge of dialling triple zero. Eventually I managed to coerce her into the car (prayer helped) and we drove back to our place, which I'm sure she now viewed as a heavily guarded, impenetrable fortress.

On another memorable (for all the wrong reasons) occasion, Ross was forced into playing reluctant bodyguard. Mum wanted to walk to the shops. He told her he'd be happy to go with her and that it really wasn't okay for her to go alone. 'Don't be ridiculous,' was her predictable reply. She broke out via the door, busting through our feeble defences, crossed the road (without looking) and began her expedition on foot. Ross followed her out and calmly explained again that he'd need to come with her, or she'd have to turn back – information not met with much avidity from Mum, to say the least. He proceeded to stand in her way. Coming from a place of sheer frustration, I'm sure, Ross was assailed by a series of punches and kicks from his very own mother-in-law. It was like an episode of *The Benny Hill Show*.

Not long after this, when trying to prevent Mum from making one of her spontaneous, speedy exits, I too bore the brunt of her new-found aggression. She launched herself towards me like a screaming banshee, pushing me off balance and sending me toppling down the front stairs. Not even the sight of her daughter laying in a crumpled heap at the foot of the steps was able to arouse a tincture of tenderness or remorse. She clambered over me to make her escape without so much as a backward glance. If I didn't know better, I'd have sworn this woman was an imposter.

Mum was also doing bizarre things, like washing the dishes with cold water and no detergent. When I mentioned that hot water and suds might be the go if we intended to avoid salmonella, she pointed to the rinsed plates and said, 'Can you see any germs on there? They're spotless!' I recalled out loud that she was the one who taught me that germs are invisible.

When I made the gentle suggestion that it might be a good idea to unstick the Post-it note that displayed her PIN number in bold writing from her credit card, she looked at me as if I'd just declared her mother wore army boots, then refused to remove it on the grounds that everyone she knows does the same thing.

I mentioned earlier that Mum had developed a reluctance to shower. When she stayed with us, this became abundantly apparent. Our spare room has an ensuite and I suggested Mum might like to have a wash and freshen up. I startled her when bringing in a towel and discovered her standing there, fully clothed, running the shower so I would *think* she was soaping up. Though it was slightly amusing, it was also eye-opening.

Soon after that, my daughter spied some bugs making their home in Mum's normally coiffured bouffant. As you can imagine, it was an uncomfortable topic of conversation to have to broach with your mother: 'Ah ... Mum ... I notice you ... er ... have quite a serious case of nits.' She vehemently renounced this insinuation, but a closer inspection revealed nothing less than an infestation.

I was racked with guilt, realising it had no doubt been one of my children who had inadvertently passed them on to their unsuspecting grandmother, maybe months before. I must pause to say how detestable these little good-for-nothing blood-suckers are and how hard to eradicate they can be. Rabbits are the traditional poster animals for breeding (if ever there was such a thing), but they've got nothing on nits! Nits could outdo a rabbit any day of the week.

I'd had plenty of experience manoeuvring a fine-toothed comb through my children's manes (which is needless to say since I had four of them) but none of those runs on the nit-removal scoreboard had prepared me to de-louse Mum. She was not happy. She did not cooperate. It was hell. Amid a tirade of acidic insults, I had to pull up stumps and concede defeat.

Fortunately, a good friend had given me the business card of a woman who made a living as a 'Nit Buster'. The card had been sitting comfortably in my wallet, waiting to be pulled out as a last resort one day. I made the necessary call, explaining to this godsend of a woman that Mum had dementia and may be a little resistant to the whole nit-busting process. As it turned out, Mum did sit still and cooperate, despite hurling occasional abuse at the beautiful and understanding soul that was the nit remover. Crisis averted.

Mum shadowed my every move that week and while normally it would have been great to spend so much time with her, I was gobsmacked by just how much she was changing. She continued to say things that were totally out of character, and although she managed to partake enthusiastically in conversations with my friends, many of them were left scratching their heads (not nit-related), wondering what she was talking about.

I now know that Mum's particular type of dementia affected a part of her brain that is the filter: the part that says, 'That's enough' and supplies the tact to be considerate of others' feelings. I was encountering an entirely new Mum, one who said it like it was. There was not a whisker of diplomacy to be found. Where once she may have walked on eggshells to preserve someone's fragile ego or searched hard for ways to encourage in the face of a seeming failure, now Mum had the subtlety of a battering ram.

Though this was hard to get used to, it did provide some comic relief. When eating at our local Italian restaurant, Mum declared aloud, well within earshot of the lovely young waitress who had just delivered it with a smile, that her pasta looked 'grey and revolting' and it tasted 'bland and disgusting'. Not only that but 'how the hell' was she supposed to eat that 'enormous, ridiculously sized mound'? You had to laugh. Around this time she also told everyone they needed a haircut and a shave (to which my girls didn't take too kindly), and let me know I needed to lose weight and that my pants made me look fat. She was on fire.

That week with Mum at our place really was illuminating. Often during the wee hours of the morning, she would wander into the girls' bedrooms looking for the toilet (is that why they call it the wee hours?). One night she tried to climb into bed with our daughter, scaring the daylights out of her, and she also wandered out the front door a couple of times in the dead of night. In the end, Ross had to sleep downstairs on the lounge, with one eye open, keeping guard.

CONSULTING THE EXPERTS

It was blatantly apparent that Mum couldn't be safe at home unless Dad was prepared to be on watch twenty-four seven. It was also apparent that he wasn't prepared to do this. Perhaps it was unfair to expect this of him; after all, it would be a massive upheaval for them both. Dad would lose his independence completely and Mum, still adamantly in denial of her snowballing deterioration, would feel like Dad was stifling her independence as well. Dad was maintaining that, on the whole, Mum was 'fine'. I knew in my heart that she needed to go into some sort of care. Ben knew it as well. It was going to be tough to convince Dad.

One night during Mum's stay at our place, in a moment of respite, I was venting my frustration and despair to some friends and asking for advice. One of my friends had been through a similar experience with her father and was able to give me the guidance no one else had so far. 'Have you had an ACAT assessment done?' she asked matter-of-factly. A what? I'd never heard of it and had no idea what she was talking about. When she explained, I wondered why on earth our Dr Gerry – admittedly a man of very few words – had failed to mention that any such thing even existed.

ACAT is an initiative of the Australian Government and stands for the Aged Care Assessment Team. It's a body that can assess the needs of an elderly person and give a recommendation for the type of care that would best suit their needs. They can visit the person at home, which was very handy because Mum wouldn't have had a bar of it if we'd had to take her to a clinic. They meet face-to-face and comprehensively assess the care needs of the individual, helping loved ones and carers to navigate the labyrinth of care options available, make informed decisions and tailor care to best fit the needs of the person in question.

Feeling nervous, like this was a devious act of espionage – a dastardly exercise in going behind Mum's back – I made an appointment for the ACAT representative to visit Mum at our place. My sister-in-law Julie came over to offer moral support, bolstering the ranks should Mum really flip out about the unexpected and, from her perspective, unwarranted visitor (not to mention my act of treason). It was an awkward wait for that all-important knock at the door. We had decided not to warn Mum of the impending visit.

Eventually, two lovely, friendly faced women fronted up, a doctor and a nurse. As expected, Mum was less than impressed. She became quite aggressive and refused to meet one-on-one with either of them. In their infinite wisdom, they suggested we wait it out. They spent some time with Julie and me, going through some basic questions about Mum's behaviour.

As they'd predicted, Mum did become less aggressive and, calmed by these consummate professionals and their gentle ways, was persuaded to cooperate. She was whisked off into another room to be questioned by the doctor before she changed her mind. If the doctor had expected a meeting with Miss Congeniality, she must have been sorely disappointed. Julie and I squirmed in our seats as Mum's louder than necessary protests echoed down the hallway. It was a relief to see that the good doctor was schooled in resilience, quite used to such a lack of cooperation from her patients. She seemed completely unfazed by Mum's tirade and pressed on with her assessment.

Once she'd resigned herself to the whole assessment thing, Mum was given a quick cognitive evaluation test, or Mini Mental Test, as it's sometimes called. Some of the questions were:

State the day, month and year. Not only did Mum have absolutely no idea of the day or date, but she didn't even know what year it was.

Draw a clock face at ten past eleven. Mum was thoroughly confused and drew an empty square.

Count backwards from one-hundred by sevens. After intense concentration and effort, Mum was able to get to ninety-three. She could go no further.

Name as many animals as you can. Now, normally Mum could give the Attenborough brothers a run for their money and was a walking encyclopaedia when it came to our friends in the animal kingdom. On this occasion, however, she struggled to name a single creature aside from 'cat' and 'dog'.

What had happened to my mother?

Mum was also given a test called the MoCA, or Montreal Cognitive Assessment, which was originally devised by Canadian Dr Ziad Nasreddine, a clever neurologist (aren't they all?) who developed his own comprehensive cognitive screening test in 1992. This test was widely acclaimed and used all over the world, but it was considered lengthy, especially if there was a high volume of patients to see. He adapted the test, bringing it down to just ten minutes without losing the essential elements needed to accurately assess cognitive function, impairment or the early stages of neurodegenerative conditions such as dementia. It was now so easy to use, here was the doctor about to administer the test to Mum in the comfort of our own home. She would be given a Memory Index Score (MIS) out of thirty, which would indicate where she was at, cognitively speaking.

The ACAT visitors were incredibly helpful and understanding. They left us with a thorough report that outlined the findings of their assessment and provided recommendations for Mum's future care and wellbeing.

Extract from the Montreal Cognitive Assessment test (MoCA).

The report from the doctor stated the following:

DIAGNOSIS

Patient has frontotemporal dementia with marked behavioural and psychological symptoms of dementia. Recent Cognitive Assessment (MoCA) score was 13/30. She displays no insight into her cognitive impairment or behavioural difficulties and their impact on her family.

REASONS FOR THE DECISION

The decision to approve you for High Level Residential Care and High Level Residential Respite Care and Home Care Level 3 & 4 has been made under section 22-1 of the Aged Care Act 1997.

FINDINGS

You were assessed as having care needs that require the provision of care and meet the other criteria for this type of care, including:

For Residential Care Permanent

Your care needs cannot be met more appropriately through other care services. In addition:

- you meet the criteria for high level residential care.

For Residential Respite Care (high)

Your care needs cannot be met more appropriately through other care services. In addition:

- you or your carer need a short-term break from your usual care arrangements, and
- you meet the criteria for high level residential care.

For a Home Care Package Level 3 or 4

Your care needs can be met appropriately through Home Care Packages. In addition:

- you prefer to remain living at home, and
- you are able to live at home with the support of a Home Care Package Level 3 or 4, and
- you meet the criteria for high level residential care.

EVIDENCE

In reaching my decision, I have considered your medical, physical, psychological and social circumstances as indicated by the following evidence:

- medical information [provided by our doctor and the ACAT doctor who had paid us a visit]
- you need help to perform daily living tasks
- you require assistance to make informed decisions about your living activities and arrangements
- you would benefit from increased social and community participation.

There it was. In black and white. Mum was no longer able to make 'informed decisions'. She could no longer 'look after' herself – let alone Dad. She did indeed need 'high care'. Her MIS score of thirteen out of thirty didn't sound too good. Further reading informed me that a score of eighteen to twenty-six would indicate mild cognitive impairment; ten to seventeen, moderate cognitive impairment; and anything under ten on the scoreboard would put you in the severe cognitive impairment category. So, let's face it, thirteen wasn't great.

Whichever way we looked at it, Mum needed care beyond what we could give her. We were faced with some big decisions. Would Mum be able to stay at home and be cared for adequately in her familiar surroundings, or would we need to look at some sort of permanent care facility? She was clearly not able to be left alone for any length of time. It was all pretty daunting. What we had to work through was nothing short of a tome, full of prospective care facilities and in-home care options – some light reading to keep me occupied for the next few weeks.

RIDING THE GUILT TRAIN

I was assailed by guilt on two levels. The first: Dad was still in Queensland, oblivious of all that was going on at home. Intensifying the betrayal, it felt like we were going behind not only Mum's back, but his too. Secondly, I felt I was unable to look after my own mother. No amount of reasoning or rationalising could take it away. I couldn't look after my own mother.

I've since met other women and men who have nursed and cared for a parent who has fallen victim to dementia. They have sacrificed a great deal, putting their own lives on hold for a time so they could be there for their loved one. This is truly an act of love, admirable and worthwhile. Many would even go so far as to say it's a duty. I felt this way and was prepared to make sacrifices. I loved my mum very much and I'd have done anything for her. This woman who had brought me into the world, suckled me at her breast and changed my nappies, who was always there with a ready bandaid if I'd skinned my knees, who mopped my brow when I was feeling sick, held my hand when I was feeling nervous, fed me, clothed me, protected me, nurtured my talents, encouraged my efforts, cuddled, kissed and loved me unconditionally ... Wasn't it my turn to look after her now?

But. There was a big but. Mum's dementia meant she needed more. She needed more than I could physically or mentally give. It was beyond me. Ben and I both struggled with this feeling of helplessness. I felt like I was monumentally letting Mum down. It was tough.

Mum had made no bones about the fact that she never wanted to live in a nursing home. There was no room for doubt about how she felt. Whenever the topic had come up in casual conversation over the years, she had made her emphatic opinion well known, in typical Mum style. In her mind, it would be hell on earth. She'd rather die than be 'shipped off'. If I asked myself whether I'd want to be 'put' in a nursing home, the answer would be categorically 'No'.

Oh, the guilt!

BATTLING THE STATUS QUO

Dad's jaunt to the Sunshine State seemed to last an eternity. I swear, had I not been so preoccupied with my mother's outlandish antics, I could've done a short course at TAFE and learnt a couple of new languages in the time it took for him to return. By the time he did touch down, he was met with great, unbridled zeal. I was brimming with new information and was ready to sprout forth with a torrent of I-told-you-so's. So much had happened while he'd been away and I was relieved we could finally show him some clear-cut evidence of what we'd been telling him for months.

In my well-meaning attempt to try to bring him up to speed with what had transpired in his absence, I may have overwhelmed him a little. Well, okay, a lot. I gave it to him in rapid-fire point form:

'The ACAT team came!

'They assessed Mum!

'The report is in and the results aren't good!

'Mum only got thirteen out of thirty in her Mini Mental test!

'Mum needs "*high care*"!

'She has to move out or a carer has to move in!

'You can't leave her alone anymore!

'We have a big book of nursing homes to look through!

'You have to read the report, Dad!

'What are we going to do ...?'

'Hang on!' Dad was not buying any of this.

Even after seeing the report and reading the recommendations, he remained resistant to admitting things had to change. My father would make a mule look like a pushover. Any discussion of Mum going into some sort of nursing home or full-time care was shut down, with Dad repeating his well-worn mantra: 'I think she'll be alright, kids.' Despite professional opinion to the contrary, Dad thought it best that Mum stay home with him and things carry on as they always had.

The sobering thing about dementia, and other degenerative diseases, for that matter, is that they are guaranteed to get worse. There's no cure on the near horizon (though hopefully one day there will be). The forecast course of this dismal ailment is hard to swallow. Dad was struggling to come to terms with the fact that things were realistically only going to get worse. If we want someone to get better badly enough, we can fool ourselves into thinking it will happen. The more we tell ourselves things are going to improve, the more we convince ourselves it's the truth. It is human nature to think there has to be a turning point. Dad was deep in denial.

There are moments in life when your hands are tied, and this was one such time. Dad wasn't going to budge and Mum was never going to admit anything was wrong. What could we do? We had to sit it out.

Dad was due to have his hip replaced in a few months' time. It would be the second time he'd be going under the knife for the same hip. He'd recently received a letter from his doctor informing him that the spare parts the surgeon had used in his previous operation had been faulty and there had been a recall – a bit like being told the airbags in your new Ford Falcon aren't up to scratch, so could you please just bring the car back in for a re-bagging? But a lot worse. What rotten luck! Or was it? Being a woman of faith, I now see this as a real turning point for Dad; there was a method in the madness – a plan was unfolding.

We knew with painful clarity that Mum wouldn't be able to stay with Ben or me while Dad was in hospital. She certainly couldn't be doing any solo stints on the home front either. I gave our wonderful ACAT nurse a call to see if she had any ideas. She gave me some great advice, suggesting we apply for three weeks' respite for Mum, in a nursing home of our choice, to allow Dad time for recovery and rehab. Once she was already in the nursing home, the best part was she could just stay on as a permanent resident if they had an available bed. This sounded like a seamless plan! Dad would see the proverbial light and Mum would already be settled in with a truckload of new friends. The transition would be as smooth as a baby's bottom.

There was just one thing we had overlooked. What if Mum point-blank refused to cooperate and wouldn't stay? We could lead this little horse to water, but she might well decide she wasn't thirsty and didn't want a drink. Then what?

JUMPING HURDLES

We finally understood what the doctor had been saying all those months before. We needed the ability to make a decision on Mum's behalf, because she was unable to make an informed, rational decision regarding her own care and wellbeing. In other words, we needed Guardianship and Power of Attorney. I tried to put myself in Mum's shoes and imagine what it would feel like to be completely stripped of your decision-making powers. It felt a little immoral. But we had to keep reminding ourselves that we were acting in her best interests, motivated by our immense love for her. We decided to apply for guardianship between Dad, Ben and me.

Two of my close friends worked together at a local nursing home – let's call it Palatial Palace – which was only a couple of years old and very swanky. Julie was also familiar with it as her nan was a resident there, enjoying the lifestyle and the staff. With it being just up the road, it seemed like the obvious choice. Dad was surprisingly on board with the plan.

I scheduled a meeting with the person in charge, and she gave Dad, Ben and me a tour of the salubrious premises. We were very impressed. It seemed more like a holiday resort than a nursing home. Each 'wing' had its own lounge room with comfy armchairs, plump pillows, the latest papers, magazines and cable TV, and its own dining room, which was equally snazzy. This place challenged my preconceived ideas of what a nursing home would be like.

My only previous peep into the private world of nursing homes had been years before, when I'd joined a bunch of fellow carollers to sing Christmas carols to the residents at a small facility in the local area. It was pretty awful, I must say. The pungent smell of urine had permeated my nostrils with every 'Glory to God in the highest' we sweetly uttered. Through pursed lips, we'd sung 'Jingle bells, (this place smells…)'. Our audience of bed-bound elderly folk looked utterly helpless and seemed to be in various stages of wasting away as they lay there appreciating our efforts with moans and smiles. I'd been consciously hoping I'd never end up in a place like that.

We had raised with Dad the possibility of Mum staying on after the respite period had elapsed, and he was prepared to at least explore the options available. The post-tour meeting was all going swimmingly, right up until the point when the nursing home representative casually mentioned the small issue of a half-million-dollar bond. Whoa! Wait a minute! Can she really have said the bond was half a million dollars? This was a major roadblock for

Dad. He barely heard anything after that clanger was dropped. Without wavering, despite Dad's loud exclamations of horror (I think he may have sworn), the patient representative explained that usually a couple would be entering the facility together and they might use the proceeds from the sale of their family home to put up as a bond. This was all well and good, but Dad was still planning to live in the family home. We ploughed on and signed the paperwork for the three weeks' respite care, figuring we'd cross the old bond bridge when we came to it.

We had a series of subsequent meetings with the staff at Palatial Palace, who assessed Mum's level of cognition to determine where she should be placed. While the nursing home was bright and shiny and not unlike a five-star hotel, visiting the dementia area on our tour of the premises had been quite confronting. One woman was lovingly rocking a doll in her arms, unwaveringly convinced it was a real baby. A couple of guys were fingerpainting with a staff member. There were loud moans and groans, seemingly emanating from the walls, and those who weren't talking to themselves animatedly, sat staring into space vacantly. Childish drawings, not unlike the ones you'd see on display in a preschool, were pinned to the walls.

Those people who, like Mum, had been afflicted with this horrible condition were cordoned off in their own locked-down area. You needed passwords, codes and a stash of keys to even get in. They were kept away from the general population, we were told, 'for their own safety and the safety of the staff and other residents'.

At that stage, I wasn't sure what that meant, though I have since learnt the hard way.

Though Mum's dementia had progressed, she was nowhere near that stage of advancement. To an outsider, she still looked and sounded relatively 'normal'. She was forgetful and talked in circles sometimes, but only those close to her were aware of the changes in her personality. Mum could comfortably converse and fit right in to any situation, dementia virtually undetectable. She was still a snappy dresser, complete with accessories and fashionable shoes; she never left home without a trendy handbag draped over her arm. She certainly didn't come across as someone with dementia. She was perky and bright and always ready with a smile.

If the dementia area had freaked me out, I figured Mum, who still believed all her marbles were firmly in place, would have an apoplectic fit should we try to move her in there. I prayed hard that they'd let her mix in with the general population, despite being tainted by her D-word diagnosis, which we had to disclose. Thankfully, after chatting with the staff, a decision was made to keep her with the general population. We could finally exhale.

FIVE-STAR DISASTER

I found myself feeling very emotional in the lead-up to Mum's stay. As I helped her pack (to avoid a repeat of the 'shoes only' debacle), the immensity of what was happening dawned on me with sad clarity. Mum was going into a nursing home. I don't think the lump in my throat left for the entire duration of her stay.

Wanting to make this little room – her temporary residence – feel like a home away from home, I set about decking it out to make it as familiar as possible. I bought a big painting of Manly Beach, Mum's old stomping ground, to adorn one of the walls of her plush private room, along with some little tables, storage for her bathroom, a fresh new doona cover and some matching towels. I also brought in a whole lot of framed photos of her family and friends, and a digital photo frame that I'd loaded up with pictures of the family. I was paranoid she would forget who we were and wanted a rolling reminder of her near-and-dear to fuel her memory. I could quiz her as the portraits faded in and out.

We were advised to bring in some familiar objects to make her feel comfortable, so I grabbed Mum's retro bedside table lamp. Purchased in the seventies, it actually is trendy now – in fact, I saw some almost identical ones in the shops recently – but it's had moments of being quite daggy over the years. Still, it was familiar to Mum, and I was hoping it would make her feel at home, the oversized orange dome-shaped shade spreading its glorious ambient light around its new abode. I hung her clothes in the wardrobe and unpacked all her toiletries. Everything was in order.

On the first day, we were welcomed into the dining room and Dad and I were invited to stay for lunch and sample some of the gourmet fare on offer. We jumped at the chance to meet some of Mum's new roomies and get a feel for the place. There was awkwardness straight away, as Mum scoffed at the dear old ladies at our table and made fun of their 'bibs'. Granted, it was strange to see fully grown adults submitting to oversized terry towelling mess-catchers being thrust over their heads without the slightest qualm or hint of embarrassment. The meal itself, though, was truly impressive, presented in various states of texture according to each individual's needs. The less dexterous of the bunch were greeted with an offering already cut into bite-sized pieces, while those lacking an incisor or two were served the same meal in puréed form. Some were spoon-fed by the caring staff. The food was delicious – far from the institutionalised tucker I was expecting.

The staff members were aware that Mum had dementia, but

the other residents were not, so it was amusing to see the puzzled looks on their faces when Mum would attempt to join in the conversation but make no sense whatsoever. They would shoot me a glance that said, 'What the ...?' But I was hardly prepared to explain Mum's condition in front of her. I valued my life too much. The residents were dear old ladies, and over the course of the weeks I learnt all their names, who their children were, the names and numbers of their grandchildren, where their husbands had served in the war, and which particular aches and pains were ailing them on any given day.

The first day had gone without a hitch, and so the next morning I pulled into the parking lot eager to learn how Mum had found her new accommodation overnight. I wasn't prepared for the scene that awaited me.

All of my efforts to turn Mum's room from a generic four-walls-and-a-bed into her own little piece of home had been meticulously dashed. Every single thing I'd set up or brought in had been dismantled. Her oversized suitcase was stuffed to the hilt and she had neatly packed up all the photo frames, stacking them efficiently in a plastic bag by the door. She had reduced all the shelves to their former flat-packed glory. They too sat stacked at the door, ready for departure, along with her groovy lamp. Every piece of clothing had been unhung. The room now stood as empty as it had been upon her arrival. She had been thorough; I'll give her that!

Mum was virtually pacing, waiting for me to walk through

the door and bring her salvation from what she still saw as an institution, despite its attempts to masquerade as a luxurious five-star resort. She hadn't been fooled and now all she desperately wanted was to go home.

As I'd cruised the halls the previous day and peered curiously into other residents' 'pieces of home', I'd seen pictures of happiness that shouted to me that they felt, if nothing else, settled. This was clearly their home now. Antique glass-fronted cabinets displayed treasured relics of bygone eras and beds were made cosier with hand-made quilts and cross-stitched pillows. Grandkids' art decorated the walls and family photos were proudly displayed. One fellow, noticing I'd been struggling to erect my flat-pack shelving sans Allen key, had introduced himself and beckoned me into his one-room abode. He had decked it out like a workshop, the walls lined with neat cabinets full of tools and knick-knacks. Handing me a couple of options to help get the job done, I marvelled at his sense of peace. He clearly had a feeling of belonging and ownership. Maybe it was naïve, but that was what I'd hoped Mum would feel too.

STEVE MCQUEEN, EAT YOUR HEART OUT (THE GREAT ESCAPE)

Unpacking and re-furnishing Mum's room became a daily occurrence for me over the next couple of weeks. No amount of reasoning could stop her relentless packing up, always done after I'd left. I would spend the first half hour of my visit re-hanging all the clothes in the wardrobe, placing things back on the shelves, re-stocking the bathroom with toiletries, putting everything back into place ... only to find, the next morning, everything packed, zipped and loaded once more. It seriously was like Groundhog Day.

My genius idea of taking the suitcase home to my place so she'd have nothing to pack backfired monumentally. Mum became obsessed with plastic bags, morphing into a bounty hunter in pursuit of these much-coveted receptacles. I'd often find her in other residents' rooms trying to coax them into upending the contents of their own plastic bags so she could score. Instead of seeing one giant packed suitcase at her door, now I became accustomed to a row of plastic shopping bags stuffed full almost to breaking with the contents of Mum's room. One day, from afar, I saw her wheeling and dealing with one of the cleaners, somehow procuring for herself a whole roll of garbage bags, which, amusingly, she then stuffed up her shirt. She feigned innocence until they dropped out on the floor and the game was up.

In order to enter or exit Palatial Palace, a security code needed to be punched into a keypad. Typically, there was a steady flow of relatives and friends coming and going through the security door each day. Mum, the Queen of Small Talk at the best of times, was still able to converse and chit-chat while keeping her dementia virtually undetectable; she decided, on this particular day, to put these skills to good use. She had begun chatting to a group of unsuspecting visitors on their way out, following them through the security door like she was slipstreaming through a carpark boom gate on someone's tail without a ticket. No one stopped her. Meanwhile, I was forty-minutes' drive away, visiting Dad at the hospital after he'd had the hip operation.

My phone rang. It was my boss, speaking in a hushed but urgent tone, insisting that he had my mother in the store with him. My workplace, a local surf shop where I work part-time (and have done since I was fifteen years old) was quite close to the Palatial Palace. At first I laughed this off. Surely he must have been mistaken. She was tucked safely away in the fancy nursing home half a kilometre up the road ... wasn't she? Oh my gosh! She'd escaped!

Our son Sam, who was incidentally also my work colleague at that time, was in the store that day and tried to talk some sense into Mum. 'It's me, Nanna. It's Sam. Are you okay? What are you doing here?' Sam was understandably rattled that his own nanna didn't recognise him, and he wasn't sure what to do. No one was! Ben, Ross and Julie were all at work in the city. My boss couldn't leave work; I was stuck so far away. What could I do? By the time I drove there, she could be anywhere!

I called my beautiful friend Keryn, who lives in the very same street as the nursing home, and in a coincidence that could only have been divinely engineered, she had been to visit Mum that morning. Keryn was there in a jiffy and found a very disoriented woman wielding a giant cake box. Mum was comforted by Keryn's familiar face and obligingly accompanied her back home. What an angel! I was so grateful.

It turns out Dad had given Mum a fifty-dollar note to pop in her wallet, much like you'd give your children if they were heading off to school camp, just in case of emergencies. A nice gesture from Dad but, let's face it, there wasn't really anywhere to spend the money. That is, of course, unless you were to slip out to the bakery and buy yourself a few dozen mini apple pies, which is exactly what Mum had done.

The staff at Palatial Palace, who I'm fairly sure were yet to discover they even had an escapee on their hands, were very red-faced and apologetic, and quick to erect multiple signs around the Palace urging visitors to 'Beware of sneaky residents trying to tailgate' (or words to that effect).

* * *

The staff were great at dealing with the elderly but not so adept with those afflicted with dementia. I'm unsure whether it was due to Mum being in with the general population and their simple forgetfulness of her condition, but they seemed quite ill-prepared to deal with her antics. Just as she had been at our place, Mum was totally fixated on going home. She was constantly devising a plan to get there and relentlessly reminded the staff of her obsession. When asked, ad nauseam, what she was doing there, when was she allowed to go home and who was picking her up, the staff would tell Mum adamantly but gently (no doubt through gritted teeth) that she wasn't going home, this was her home now and she was staying put. Full stop.

You can imagine how well this went down. So well, in fact, that on one occasion, Mum gave one of the nurses her best left hook. Our whole family was called in, informed of the full extent of our delinquent mother's crime, and told in the kindest words possible that once Mum's stint of respite was over there wouldn't be a long-term place for her. It was like being back in the school Principal's office. So, Mum had punched a nurse. But it wasn't her fault! Didn't they know she had dementia, and this was completely out of character?

COPYBOOK BLOTTED

Effectively, Mum had been kicked out of Palatial Palace and had completely blotted her copybook . Unfortunately, any other nursing home we approached would be privy to the rather scathing report that had accompanied my mother on her way out through those salubrious doors. Words so completely opposite to Mum's normally bubbly, congenial character, like 'violent', 'aggressive' and 'anti-social', littered this document we were forced to produce at every new doorway. It was a stumbling block of epic proportions.

We were right back at square one. Once again, we thumbed through the giant book of nursing homes and facilities. Now we were not only looking for one we liked; we were looking for one that would take a feisty, female, seventy-something Muhammad Ali. We had our work cut out for us. As we set about making a few enquiries, some knocked us back over the phone, citing all their good reasons for rejecting Mum, including the fact that the entry of someone aggressive into their 'settled' little dementia units would really just upset the balance. They weren't prepared to take the risk. Damn that report!

To add to this, Dad had been recuperating from his operation and was now continuing his recovery at a rehab hospital. With plenty of time to ponder his and Mum's predicament, he had once again successfully convinced himself that he could look after Mum after all, perhaps with a little in-home care. They'd be fine. He was sure. It was so frustrating.

His hip pocket featured heavily in the equation too. While Ben and I were upset that it had come down to money, I guess it was understandable, given Dad was now retired and any money he and Mum had in savings had to last for the rest of their lives. I know Mum and Dad had envisaged spending these savings sailing into a Pacific sunset or travelling around the globe together. This was a far cry from what they'd had in mind. It must be frightening to watch your savings get chewed up by completely unforeseen circumstances. All Dad's ruminating had led him to this good excuse not to upset the applecart. As far as finding full-time residential care for his wife was concerned, his feet were well and truly cold.

As part of Dad's rehab process, a meeting was scheduled with a social worker to assess how care would continue once he returned home. It was very fortuitous that I happened to be visiting when this wonderful woman was meeting with him. The discussion turned to who would be at home when Dad was discharged from hospital, and he chirped up to say his wife would be there. I honestly think Dad had convinced himself Mum was up to looking after him and nursing him back to good health upon his return. In a timely moment, I was able to chime in and inform her of the real story, the reality of Mum's condition, and to discuss with her all that had gone before. The social worker inquired about Mum's MoCA test score and when I revealed to her the solemn results, she was absolutely dumbfounded at what Dad was contemplating. She strongly encouraged him to rethink the options. I wanted to hug her! What an answered prayer. She really was a godsend!

The social worker came back several more times to talk things through with Dad and he seemed to respect her professional opinion. Though the information was just what we had already told Dad, nothing new, she seemed to be able to slice through his denial and open his eyes.

Dad came out of hospital with a new hip and a new attitude.

* * *

To add a little more stress to an already stressful situation, it was brought to our attention that the legislation in Australia surrounding aged care fees was about to change. Certain 'reforms' would come into force from 1 July of that year, affecting means testing – specifically, what was and wasn't to be included as an asset when calculating your fee schedule. There was a base daily fee to cover meals, accommodation and general care and then, on top of that, was another fee based on your assets and ability to afford it. Mum and Dad had properties and other investments up their sleeves. Suffice to say, it was going to cost significantly more for Mum to live in any aged care facility after July. Annoyingly, it was already June when this information came to light.

Julie, Dad and I began our Nursing Home Tour Extraordinaire. We left no stone unturned and saw the gamut of options available. Mum came along to a few homes too, which was slightly awkward, given she saw herself as being in perfect health, mentally and otherwise. There were fancy ones with grand pianos, chandeliers and happy hours every night at five o'clock. Some homes were hideous and reminiscent of my carol-singing days, thick with stench. Others were sterile and devoid of atmosphere – more like a hospital than a home. At one place, we witnessed a poor lady being literally dragged back – a different nurse on each of her four limbs, her skinny, half naked body hanging down like a hammock – after an attempted escape on hands and knees. Her shrill howling echoed around the tired walls. Even just witnessing it made me feel like I was violating this poor soul's privacy. It certainly wasn't an environment to ever wish upon a loved one.

Knowing how much Mum disliked nursing homes and loved being at home, we explored the possibility of in-home care. It would be ideal: Mum could stay in her familiar environment while still getting all the care she needed. Dad could be with her, which would make the transition easier on him too. Research[1] has shown that the onset of symptoms can be delayed if the person suffering from dementia is able to stay in familiar surroundings. Ben and I explored this option with hopeful rigour.

Many in-home care providers had waiting lists longer than my arm. Eventually we were able to meet with a very lovely, caring woman (she was in the right profession), who tried hard to find us a cost-effective in-home care option. In the end, though, we discovered it was going to be even more expensive than residential care – a clear concern for Dad. We also realised Mum needed round-the-clock care, which they just couldn't offer. All the while we had to remember, beggars can't be choosers. Mum had a rap sheet now and time was running out. Though those already residing in care homes were safe from the price rise, if we wanted to beat the scheduled hike in fees for those entering care for the first time, we needed to hurry.

In the interim, Dad had decided to take Mum away to the Gold Coast for a couple of weeks, staying in their Surfers Paradise holiday unit. Arriving at the airport, they checked their bags and headed for the security check. Mum and Dad have both had various body parts upgraded and replaced over the years, so setting off the alarms when going through customs is par for the course for them. Mum caused a loud beep as she sauntered through the scanner and was recalled for another go through. Dad tried to explain that it was Mum's titanium hip raising the alarm, but Mum argued black and blue that she had never, under any circumstances, gone under the knife in such a fashion. A loud argument ensued, escalating when Dad explained that his wife had dementia.

'What are you bloody well talking about, Tony?' Mum bellowed. 'I've had no such operation. You're being completely ridiculous!'

Poor Dad.

Mum hadn't been drinking in respite, but once she was back with Dad, he'd encouraged her to have a glass of wine over dinner and she'd slipped back into old habits. After all, this was their usual pattern. It was what she normally would have done. Dad had failed to stop and think that this may not have been the wisest choice, given that his wife was no longer 'normal'. One drink turned to several one night, and the evening concluded with Mum being unable to walk and having to be carried by Dad and the friendly publican all the way back to their unit. Even Dad now recognised that something had to be done.

* * *

The Nursing Home Tour Extraordinaire had just about exhausted its options. After all our seeking, and virtually at the eleventh hour, we thanked God for his faithfulness: we finally had a breakthrough. Just one week from the dreaded deadline, we found somewhere willing to take Mum. It was a facility that was entirely for dementia sufferers, so there was no such thing as the 'general population' distinction there had been at Palatial Palace. There was a huge outdoor area with herb gardens, bird baths and little pathways winding through gardens and trees. There were shady areas to sit among the birds and plenty of space to wander. If I'm honest, the decor was a little dated and daggy, but Mum's would-be room was bright and freshly painted, and it even had a little balcony overlooking a leafy garden. It was the happy medium between Palatial Palace and the sterility of a hospital environment.

We met with the manager and she was able to fast-track the registration process for us so we could meet the 1 July deadline. On 30 June, just in the nick of time, Mum moved in.

BEGINNINGS AND ENDINGS

There's no doubt it was confronting walking into this place, knowing that Mum would be moving in. The small dementia ward at Palatial Palace was one thing, but this was a whole new kettle of fish. The facility, being entirely dedicated to those with dementia was a very different atmosphere to the quiet, well-behaved general population of Palatial Palace. Mum was still a long way from where most of these dear residents were at, their slide into cognitive oblivion well-advanced. At only seventy-three, she was a spring chicken compared to most of the population, some of whom looked to be just a shade under triple digits. Mum cupped her hand over her mouth and leant in close, her eyes wide, whispering, 'What on earth is going on here?'

We bought Mum a new TV for her room, hung some pictures, unpacked and put her clothes away. A generous friend gave us a fantastic remote-controlled recliner chair, which we popped in the corner, and I bought some colourful cushions to brighten the place up a bit. On the surface, it all seemed fine. I smiled for Mum and tried to reassure her that things would be okay here. 'What a great room, Mum! You'll love it here! The gardens are so pretty!'

My words had the dual purpose of trying to convince us both they were true.

On the outside, I was desperately trying to keep it all together, but inside I was nothing short of devastated; anguish writhed behind my cool, calm facade. I felt as if I would either throw up or burst into tears at any moment. My throat was thick with knots and my eyes were glassing over. I thought of my family home. Our family home. The house that Mum had lovingly transformed into a home for us all. A house that still stood full of Mum's beautiful things, Mum's exquisite taste, her personality embedded in every corner. She was the one who had lovingly decorated it, chosen the artworks that adorned the walls, picked out the quirky knick-knacks that we so loved. She was the one who had filled the shelves with the books she'd read. Her wardrobe was still packed with her colourful outfits and shoes. Her pots and pans lined the kitchen cupboards. Everything was just where she'd left it. The garden was fragrant with freesias she'd hand-planted from bulbs collected from Grandma's. It was the place she'd called home for forty-nine years. The stark reality hit me right then. Mum would never again go home. Dad would live alone. Mum and Dad's was now just Dad's. It was heartbreaking.

No doubt these emotions are familiar to anyone who has

experienced the death of a parent. The cruel reality of dementia is that even though your parent is still alive, it is as if they are not. The person you knew and loved is gone. The death of a parent or loved one, whether sudden and unexpected or painfully anticipated, brings with it a raw and agonising finality. Your grief has a start date; a chapter has closed. When dementia is involved, there's a very real grieving that takes place, but there's no single point when you realise they have actually gone. The edges are blurred around where they cease to be themselves and become someone else entirely. It creeps up behind you like a balaclava-clad thief stalking around in the dark, until suddenly the lights flash on and you realise this stealthy enemy – dementia – has stolen your parent right out from under your nose. Not only has it stolen who they are, but it's stripped you of the precious relationship you shared with them. Physically, they are still present. You can cuddle them, hold their hand, sit with them. There is a familiarity in their smile, in their touch, in their voice. Ultimately, though, they are here but not here. Your interactions will forevermore, cruelly, be altered.

We were heading into unmapped territory, in the dark, on an unsealed, one-way road – and the brakes were failing. We had so many preconceived ideas about this disease, but had no idea of what sort of timeline we were looking at. Would Mum remember us next week, next year? There was no answer. It was terrifying.

* * *

Hazel Hawke, the much-loved ex-wife of our larrikin former Prime Minister, the late Bob Hawke, had recently and sadly succumbed to her dementia, passing away around the time Mum had started to display her changing behaviours. Hazel Hawke was a spokeswoman for Alzheimer's disease and gained the sympathy of her fellow Australians when she was interviewed candidly on national TV about what was happening to her. She, unlike my mother, had a real awareness of what was going on. She was fully cognisant that she was not always fully cognisant. She knew emphatically what she had fallen victim to. In light of what was happening to Mum, it was fascinating to hear her eloquently articulating her experience of having dementia. This was the complete antithesis of Mum who, like a child who is nodding off mid-sentence while insisting they are 'not tired', aggressively attested to her immaculate mental health, despite its very apparent demise.

Now armed with information about dementia in its various forms, we understand that Hazel Hawke's Alzheimer's disease had vastly different symptoms and characteristics to Mum's behavioural variant frontotemporal dementia, but one of Dad's favourite catchphrases at the time was: 'Why can't your mother be like Hazel Hawke and just admit she has dementia?' It would have been a lot easier.

SETTLING IN

Unlike Palatial Palace, this new place, let's call it Leafy Lodge, discouraged its residents from spending time alone in their rooms. This worried me slightly, as I'd imagined Mum might like to come up to the comfort of her own room when things (read: 'people') became a little overwhelming in the common rooms with the other residents. She could go to her room to get away from it all for a time, kick back in her comfy recliner rocker and watch a midday movie or two.

Whenever I went to visit her, I'd try to remove her from the masses and whisk her away to her private oasis. It was clear, though, that she wasn't even the slightest bit interested in watching television. This, from a woman who had once thrived on stretching out on the lounge in front of the box, immersing herself in a decent doco or drama in her down time.

Dad was both perplexed, as he likes a good veg out in front of the tele as much as anyone, and frustrated, because the remote control in Mum's room kept disappearing. He was convinced someone was stealing it and if it had been in his power, he would have ordered a Royal Commission into the whereabouts of that damn remote control. Remote Controlgate. Dad kept up regular interrogations of the staff, who continually professed their innocence, while I obediently and repeatedly replaced the said missing item with 'universal' models, at Dad's insistence. No matter what we tried, they just kept walking. Mum remained completely oblivious to what we were even searching for.

The plot thickened when the remote control for the recliner chair also vanished. This was not as easily replaced and took away all enjoyment for my teenage kids, who loved nothing more than to go from a lying position to a standing position in record time, gleefully ejecting one another from the chair's clutches, whenever they visited Mum. Unfortunately, the final button pushed before the remote went missing, placed the chair in the Bolt Upright position, a position belying the recliner's very name and most certainly not conducive to comfort. A position it shall sadly remain in forevermore.

Whether or not there were thieves at work in the whole Remote Controlgate scandal is yet to be confirmed, but there was definitely some 'sharing' of possessions going on among the residents. It was a shock to arrive one day and see Joan decked out in one of Mum's unmistakably stylish outfits. Mum also began sporting a rather shaggy looking pink cardigan that was clearly not hers.

Surprisingly, her name had been dutifully sewn inside the collar! Many times after that, Mum appeared in fancy, new, never before seen earrings and necklaces, and various other pieces of newly 'acquired' apparel.

It was very amusing to find a lovely family photo beside Mum's bed one day – though alarming, too, as the handsomely dressed ensemble gathered within the frame was not her family. She also had a beautiful picture of a couple of good-looking strangers on their wedding day. I asked Mum if she could identify the happy couple, but she had absolutely no idea who they were or what she was doing with their happy snap. The funniest thing was, she saw nothing at all strange in the fact that this picture of two complete strangers was taking pride of place on her bedside table.

BIG FAT LIARS

Mum was still as fixated as ever with going home. Just as she had done in respite, she'd pack that big old suitcase every day and lug it all the way from her room up the hill, down the gentle slope to reception, determined she was checking out. With machine-gun-like incessancy, Mum would pester the staff about where Dad was, how she was getting home, who was picking her up and so on. It never stopped. Whenever I popped in to visit, I'd spy Mum from the other side of the room, verbally harassing some poor member of the team. Their patience was virtuous.

It was obvious that the staff had been trained well in what to expect from and how to deal with dementia sufferers. Instead of becoming frazzled or giving pat answers to Mum's persistent quizzing as to why she couldn't go home, the staff were gentle and comforting. Every afternoon, just before dinner, my mother would plod down to the dining room, fully packed and exasperated, asking what was happening and 'Where was Tony?'

Very calmly, they would tell her that the taxi had been ordered and would be there in an hour. Mum needed only to go inside and have dinner and, before she knew it, she'd be climbing aboard her ride out of there. Home with Tony in no time flat. At this news, Mum would beam back at the beautiful staff member and cooperatively venture inside for her evening meal. While she ate, the staff would return her bag to her room and quietly unpack its contents, so Mum was none the wiser. After a relaxing dinner, she would retire for the night, completely oblivious to what had gone on only an hour before.

This worked a treat but ... they'd lied. Up until that point, I'd been at pains to be as honest as possible with Mum. I wanted to convince her she had a problem. I wanted her to admit she needed care and validate our decision to institutionalise her. I wanted her to know how much we loved her and wanted the best for her. I wrote little notes to her explaining what was going on, which I would leave in her room.

Dear Mum,

A few months ago you had a brain scan and it showed some of your brain had started to atrophy or shrink. We now know you have dementia, even though you don't think you do. I know it's hard to understand and this is all really confusing for you but being here is the best option for you and you'll get all the care and medical attention you need. We will visit you ALL the time.

*You know we love you very, very dearly and would only ever
want the best for you.*

Love you lots and lots and lots, Mum.
See you soon,
Sarah xoxoxo

I needed her to concede she had dementia. I realised I was just like
Dad; I wanted her to be like Hazel Hawke. To Mum I must have
sounded ridiculous. For the most part, she'd screw up my notes
and throw them into the wastepaper basket. There was one that
she kept in her handbag and pulled out to read every now and
then. Upon reading it, a scowl would stretch across her face, before
she'd promptly stuff it back in her bag, muttering, 'What a load of
rubbish', or something to that effect.

It felt so wrong to lie to her and I struggled to wrap my morals
around the whole idea of making stuff up. I despise dishonesty and
the truth is paramount to me, but here I was faced with this dilemma,
not knowing whether to twist the truth to make things easier for
Mum or to rigidly maintain honesty at all times. There was an
obvious change in Mum's mood when she was served this completely
fabricated story. I witnessed first-hand her anxiety melting away as
she took false comfort in an imaginary taxi that would never turn up.
It soothed her like the cold, hard facts never could have.

One of the gorgeous Leafy Lodge staff members had developed
a standard reply to Mum's constant questioning regarding Dad's

whereabouts. She would say, 'Jeannie, remember I told you Tony's at the State of Origin game with Ben?' Despite the fact that it was the middle of summer and everybody knew State of Origin was only played in winter, Mum would fall for this story hook, line and sinker. No matter what time of year or what time of day (or night) it was, this alibi stood up to the test; Mum was satisfied that Dad was safely ensconced, with their son, in a grandstand at the stadium watching a state vs state (mate vs mate) game of rugby league. Every day it was the same spurious excuse and every day she believed it.

Another favourite was to tell Mum that Tony was 'at the gym'. Since Dad did make daily visits to his shrine of fitness, this excuse was plausible. To the ubiquitous inquiries of 'Where am I? Why am I here?' we would lie through our teeth, saying that she was just there for a couple of days while Dad was at the hospital/away on business/at a body corporate meeting in Queensland ... Choose your own adventure. If she thought her stay in the home was temporary, the blow was softened.

It didn't feel right to be spinning her these lies, but the truth only made her angry and exasperated. I tried to find a happy medium. To Mum's desperate interrogations of when I'd next be there to take her home, for example, I'd choose between answering honestly ('I'll be back in a couple of days to see you, but you'll have to stay here.') and giving the more ambiguous yet palatable answer ('I'll be back very soon to see you.'). I may have been quibbling over semantics, but it made me feel better.

MEMORY MATTERS

Though Mum's dementia was clearly progressing, she could still easily converse, and she could shower, toilet and dress herself. She was the new kid on the block and it was clear she was still the most 'with it' mentally. One of Mum's fellow residents was a long way down the track. She didn't look very old – maybe in her early sixties – but she would stare vacantly at you with her big blue eyes and mumble incoherently to no one in particular. With her hair worn in a youthful ponytail, she would wander around aimlessly and then perform a random act, like calling out with her arms held aloft before sitting on the floor abruptly. Let's call her Sally. For Dad, Sally was a benchmark. He often commented, 'Well, at least your mother is nowhere near as bad as Sally!' A hollow consolation, but Sally's worsening condition brought comfort to Dad.

At this stage, Mum's short-term memory took a real dive. She'd forget what had just been said within seconds. It was incomprehensible. It was almost comical. We could certainly empathise with Nemo. Whenever Mum would ask a question hot on the heels of the answer I'd just given her for the exact same question, I'd find myself thinking, Are you serious?

On one occasion, when Mum had come to our place for a visit, she was sitting at our kitchen table while the washing machine in the adjacent laundry was in full flight, loudly shuddering in the throes of its fervent spin cycle.

'What's that sound, Sam?' she inquired of our eldest son.

'Oh, it's just the washing machine, Nanna, it will be finished soon,' he told her.

Seconds later, with the same curious tone, Mum repeated, 'What's that sound, Sam?'

He stayed measured and informed her again that it was just the washing machine. It would be finished soon.

She then asked a third time, a fourth, a fifth and a sixth, each time as if for the first time, in the same questioning tone. Sam, bless his patient heart, continued to answer her in the same way, despite his frustration. Mum asked thirty times what that noise was, and thirty times Sam responded that it was 'Just the washing machine, Nanna.' It would have been easier to turn it off!

To get her out and about, whenever I'd visit Mum I'd take her to a nearby cafe, which had a beautiful fountain in the foyer outside it. The first time she saw the fountain, Mum was enchanted, reacting with an open-mouthed declaration of its beauty. Two days later, when we visited again, she responded in the exact same way, as if seeing it for the very first time. The following week, it was as fresh and new to her as a brand-new sunrise, and she exclaimed with her usual, 'Oh, it's beautiful!' all over again. Over the next few months, whenever we'd go there we'd say, '*Wait* for it ...' and sure enough, the fountain would predictably, once again, be admired for its magnificence.

* * *

Still coming to grips with the depth of his wife's rapid short-term memory loss, Dad relished in giving her his specialty pop quizzes. He fired questions at her that she was never going to be able to answer.

'How many grandchildren do you have, Jeannie?

'What are Sarah's kids' names?

'Who are Ben's kids?

'Do you remember our address?

'What year is it?

'When's my birthday?

'What year did we get married?'

Whether Mum responded with silence or aggression, it was obvious to us all that the answers just weren't there. Like dew in the morning sun, or chocolate left unclaimed and unattended in our fridge, they had disappeared without a trace. It was futile. Dad would shake his head in disbelief and reiterate how incredible it was that she couldn't even name her own grandchildren. But these were not the right questions to ask.

Since the diagnosis was established, from the moment the D-word was uttered, we'd had an overriding fear that we couldn't shake. It was a fear that stalked us relentlessly, a fear that kept us up at night, a fear that we didn't even want to say out loud. The fear of the inevitable: *One day, we'll walk into her room and she won't know who we are.*

It was a day I knew was coming, a dread I tried to suppress on a daily basis. Each visit's mantra: *So far, so good.*

Although Mum might not always have remembered our names at that point, there was a definite recognition that darted across her face when our eyes met. She'd spot us across the room and her face would light up like a sparkler on cracker night. Clutching tightly to her handbag, she would make a beeline for us before begging us to take her home. It was heartwrenching and heartwarming at the same time.

WOE IS ME

I must admit, I felt somehow cheated. Mum's dementia was the enemy, there's no doubt about that, but it was easy to put a selfish twist on it and make it all about me; all about us and what we'd been robbed of.

There was one particular day when this really came to the fore. I had gone to visit Mum and had taken her to the cafe for a bite to eat. Beside us, a couple of siblings sat enjoying a cup of tea and a sandwich with their elderly mother, who happened to be wheelchair bound. Conversation with my mum had become more and more difficult, so there were plenty of lulls and pregnant pauses going on at our table. Eavesdropping was not only tempting, it was downright unavoidable (I'm sticking with that excuse, anyway).

As the conversation between these table-neighbours of ours ebbed and flowed, they chatted freely about their children, their mother seeming to delight in hearing tales of her grandchildren's exploits. The talkative siblings spoke of their jobs and colleagues and the issues each of them was facing. They would offer one another advice and a spot of encouragement here and there. They chin-wagged about current affairs, politics, television shows and music. It was a lovely morning tea for this little family group whose admiration, care and love for one another was obvious.

I should have been happy for them, but instead I found myself burning with jealousy. What I would have given to have been able to sit down with Mum and Ben like this and talk our little hearts out! Oh, how I would have loved to recount our latest stories to Mum, to boast about what the kids had been up to, for her to puff with pride like only a grandmother can. How I'd have loved to hear her take on the upcoming election or the latest episode of *Survivor*. It would have been great to ask her advice on what to do with four kids who, despite daily reminders, continued to leave their wet towels in a heap on the floor. What had she done with us? Would banning towels altogether and forcing them to dry off with a single Kleenex be too harsh? All these things, I would have loved to hear from Mum. The lady at the next table may not have had the use of her legs but her brain was intact, sharp as a tack.

I spoke to God in my head, asking, 'Why her brain, Lord? You could've taken any number of less vital body parts, but why take her brain, the essence of her? It's not fair!'

The thing about comparing yourself to others is you don't always know the full story. It's not a healthy practice and one I have tried, conscientiously, to avoid. For all our own troubles, there is always someone worse off than us. This isn't always easy to remember. Like rebuking your children for not eating their veggies and wasting food by bringing to mind for them the starving millions in other countries who would do anything to eat just one of those delicious little peas they have rejected, it is something that needs constant repeating. We all need to be deliberately conscious of what we have to be thankful for. I have to remain grateful for all the wonderful years we were able to enjoy with Mum and her fully functioning, intact mind.

BETWEEN A ROCK
AND A HARD PLACE

When Mum was in Palatial Palace, my daily visits were motivated by my strong sense of duty and obligation. I was compelled to check on how she was doing and to see that we'd made the right decision. Partly out of guilt, mostly out of love. I desperately wanted it all to work out. Now that Leafy Lodge was her new home, visiting Mum came with a whole new set of challenges. For the most part, visiting her wasn't pleasant. Adjusting to the dementia-fuelled behaviours of Mum's housemates – less than conventional to say the least – was enough on its own without Mum's constant aggression and questioning about why she was there.

Around this time, people often asked me how Mum was going and whether she was 'settled'. I didn't have the heart to tell them the half of it. She was colossally, staggeringly and unequivocally *un*settled. The word that comes to mind to best describe her state of being at that time is 'restless'. She was restless and agitated. When she saw me walk through the door, her expression was one of impatient relief. 'Well, it's about time you got here! Let's go home. Are you okay to drive me home?'

At other times, she would explain that she wasn't sure where Dad was, so 'would I be kind enough to do her a big favour and drive her home?' After six months of visiting, it astounded me that Mum still didn't know she had moved in there. I would show her to her room and let her see her own belongings to prove it, but she vehemently disputed her residency being anywhere other than our family home.

One of the preconceived ideas people often have about dementia is that it's harder for the relatives than it is for the actual sufferer. This may be so in some cases, depending on the type of dementia in question, but in our experience, this certainly didn't ring true. Mum seemed to be going through an excruciating period of inner turmoil. Her world had been turned upside down. She was not at peace, and that was torture for her.

Although she couldn't articulate it, Mum knew something was very wrong. Every fibre of her being was fighting this unwinnable war against the unknown enemy that had encamped around her rational mind and was closing in, snatching any remaining powers of reason or understanding. As swiftly as a seagull might whisk a hot chip from your hand, just as you are about to tuck in to your seaside fish and chips, leaving you robbed of the soft, salty goodness you so eagerly anticipated, dementia was stealing Mum's future. Of course, this was not how anybody expected things to pan out, least of all Mum. Something deep down in her was rebelling; against what, she wasn't sure.

Mum also became extremely unpredictable around this time. On a visit to her room, for instance, I pointed out the clothes hanging in her wardrobe, as proof that she did indeed reside in this facility. When she asked me how they came to be there, I explained that I had driven to her house, taken them from her wardrobe, and then brought them there and hung them up. Her response? 'Oh, darling, did you do that just for me? You drove all the way there and back? That is just so lovely of you, Sarah darling. Thank you!'

The very next day, when once again going through the motions of showing Mum that she did actually have her own room and a bed there, she asked me the same question and I gave her the exact answer I had given the previous day. This time, she responded with: 'How dare you! How dare you go to my house – my room – without asking me! How dare you take things out of my wardrobe without my permission! You little [insert expletives].'

It was awful. She was up and down like a yo-yo. Even when I thought I knew just what to say, she'd react as unpredictably as a high-pressure hose with no one holding it.

I felt so guilty for feeling this way but, realistically, visiting Mum was a chore and definitely not something I looked forward to. On the contrary, it was something I dreaded. She wouldn't ever remember I'd been anyway, so I felt like I was wasting my time. What was the point? A deeply embedded sense of obligation, love and loyalty told me I needed to be there and kept me going back. In my heart of hearts, I knew I couldn't stay away.

It was important to see my mother, that I knew, but my mere presence seemed to unsettle her even more, her agitation and stress levels rising noticeably as soon as I walked into the room. Leaving was incredibly hard too. She'd plead to come with me and, ironically, would call out to me as I was leaving, 'Don't forget about me!' It was so emotionally taxing, some weeks I avoided visiting at all. I would fight tears the whole time I was there and erupt into sobs the minute I returned to my car.

Taking someone with me was always easier. Whenever possible, I would meet Dad or Ben there and we'd find safety in numbers as we escorted Mum to lunch or morning tea. Sometimes many visits would go by without me being able to raise even a flicker of a smile from Mum and not for want of trying. Ben, on the other hand, always seemed to be able to get Mum giggling. It was so refreshing to see the way the two of them related. Mum would often erupt in hysterical laughter at something Ben had said or done and it would be infectious, all of us grabbing our sides, tears of joy on our cheeks.

The ridiculously early dinner time of 5 pm made it hard for Ross to accompany me, so I'd often take one or more of the kids with me to see their nanna. Before and after each visit, I felt compelled to reminisce about the 'real' Nanna, recalling lots of good times and fun memories of the kids hanging out with her. I'd apologise in advance for Mum's un-Nanna-like behaviour. I was absolutely paranoid about them forgetting who Mum was – who she really was. This was not how I wanted them to remember my darling mum. I was tempted not to bring them to visit at all, so as not to taint their picture of their nanna, to dent those precious memories or unravel the rich tapestry of her, woven over the course of their lives.

When a loved one passes away, memories of them, now finite, need to stay locked in a time capsule, preserved forever in our minds, suspended from decay like a peach in a Mason jar at the Royal Easter Show. We need to incessantly revisit those memories, lest they start to fade.

With dementia, though, beautiful memories from the past can so easily be distorted by what's going on in the present. The two strands of memory twist and intertwine, becoming indistinguishable from one another and forming an identikit version of a person, hardly recognisable as the one you have known and loved for so long. I was desperately trying to keep those strands separate. It was almost as if I believed that by keeping the kids away, their recollections of their nanna would remain true to who she was. Any merging of the two versions of Mum – pre- and post-dementia – would muddle their memories and change their fundamental perception of who she was. My constant prayer is that they will never forget what their nanna was like before this affliction invaded the sanctity of her grey matter and changed her irrevocably.

Each of our children reacted differently as they watched Mum's rapid deterioration. They had their own coping mechanisms, dealing with it in their own ways. However you look at it, it isn't easy to watch the matriarch of the family fade away, and it requires a great deal of stoicism not to fall apart at each meeting. At the time of Mum's diagnosis, Sam was nineteen, Molly was seventeen, Toby was fourteen and Maisy was just eight. Molly, who has a naturally caring and sunny disposition, would always try to rouse a smile from Mum and ask her how she was feeling. My sweet Toby was the most visibly distressed and found it the hardest to come to terms with his nanna's new personality. Whenever he knew I'd been to see her, he'd always take the time to ask how I was going and make enquiries as to the state of my wellbeing. Sam, who has always been a sensitive soul, had been shaken ever since the day of the 'great escape' when Mum, coming face-to-face with her own grandson, hadn't even recognised him. Being the youngest, Maisy has seen the most of Mum in care, often coming with me to visit her, and unfortunately her memories of her nanna are not as well-rooted and established as the older kids'. Sadly, I fear it is this 'new' version of Mum that she will remember and carry with her into the future.

REACHING FOR SPEECH

One of the major characteristics of behavioural variant frontotemporal lobe dementia, as opposed to Alzheimer's or other forms of dementia, is its effect on the speech of the sufferer. Given Mum's propensity for language and love of all things verbal, it seemed particularly cruel that this was where it would strike. When dementia originates in the frontal lobes of the brain, there is a gradual loss of the ability to speak or understand language. Like petals drying up and falling one by one from an exquisite rose, words began to slip from Mum's vocabulary. It was as if she had a limited supply and had to choose the ones from a meagre selection that best fitted the situation at hand. When trying on some pants, for instance, and finding they billowed down, gathering on the floor below her, completely concealing her feet and ankles, she was searching for the word 'long', to say, 'They're too long.' We both had a chuckle at just how long they were, but Mum struggled to articulate the problem. Apparently finding that the word 'long' was no longer in her diminishing repertoire, she spurted out that the pants were 'too bottom'! Strangely, I knew what she meant.

This kind of situation happened quite regularly. One day we were going for a coffee and when I explained where our destination was, Mum pointed heavenward and referred to it as 'The up one'. She would mean to say, 'I'll be back in a minute', but instead would claim she'd be back in an 'inch'. She must have known some sort of measurement word was required but couldn't quite call to memory the one she needed.

Another time when we were out, a glimmer of recognition came across Mum's face when she thought she saw someone she knew. Rather than saying, 'I thought she looked familiar,' Mum managed: 'I thought she liked her.' Again, I knew what she meant. It felt like a giant game of charades. I surprised myself by rising to the challenge more often than not, successfully deciphering the true meaning of Mum's cryptic mutterings. It was obvious that this groping in the dark for words was frustrating for her, though I doubt she was always aware of the inappropriateness of her chosen words.

Finding a topic of conversation was fraught. Navigating the landmines of taboo subjects left little other than the current barometric pressure or outside air temperature to ruminate over. 'What are those clouds doing out that window? Gee, the sky is blue today. Do you think it might rain this afternoon?' We couldn't talk about Dad, as that only stirred up anxiety about where he was, why he wasn't there, when he'd be back ... We couldn't really talk about the kids because, as Dad's pop quizzes had determined, Mum struggled to remember them by name. If I tried talking about Ben and Julie and their family, it was the same. It would either make her anxious, or her extreme vagueness would mean the whole, one-sided conversation was just me explaining over and over again who everyone was and what on earth I was talking about. I couldn't ask about what she had been doing because she had no recollection.

Leafy Lodge regularly took the residents on little excursions and outings, which was great. Dad would often arrive to visit Mum and be told by the staff all about an outing Mum had been on that very morning, only to find that she had absolutely no memory of it. Whether it was lunch at the club, a morning at the beach, a picnic in the park or a trip to a gallery, Mum would remain adamant that she had been firmly planted right there at the nursing home, not budging from that spot for the entire day.

Obviously current affairs were off the table for discussion, as were stock market prices, the current state of the Aussie dollar and celebrity gossip. Normally Mum was proudly abreast of the latest celebrity developments – 'People, Places and Faces', as Ben and I used to call it. She could tell you which Hollywood A-lister had either married or split from another Hollywood A-lister; she'd know who dazzled at a recent award ceremony or what ridiculous name some famous couple had encumbered their new-born with. But as dementia tightened its grip, and no matter how many gossip mags I brought for us to peruse over lunch in an attempt to fill the growing, pregnant pauses between us, it all seemed to draw a blank now. She could tell neither a Pitt from a Depp nor a Kardashian from a Minogue. Another topic of conversation down the gurgler.

All the normal things family members (or anyone, for that matter) would converse about were now unavailable. Mum's hearing difficulties had only worsened – a hearing aid out of the question now since she would most certainly misplace it – and this, coupled with our lack of topics to chat about, made communication a challenge, to say the least. Even small talk, in which Mum usually excelled, was tough.

Mercifully, our favourite spot for coffee had a large tropical fish tank and an aviary of finches. I made a point of sitting near these mesmerising creatures whenever possible, as they offered us something to look at. Pointing at the fish and chatting incessantly, I'd try to elicit some interest from Mum. Occasionally it would work. She'd point back and state the colour of the fish but would often say 'green' when she meant 'blue' or 'black' when she meant 'yellow'. Words were packing their bags and exiting Mum's brain, leaving clouds of dust in their trail.

Before her diagnosis, Mum and I would often chat about our latest reading material, swapping books to discuss in our own little book club, but Mum's capacity for reading began to diminish from quite early on in her dementia. I noticed she had a novel on her bedside table for weeks, but the bookmark never seemed to move from one visit to the next. When I asked how the book was going, she couldn't even give me a broad synopsis. Though she could still read, she'd lost her ability to concentrate for the lengthy periods required to read a book.

Something I found both amusing and sad at the same time was the way Mum would read aloud every piece of writing she laid her eyes on. Be it a menu, a street sign, a label on a packet of biscuits or a banner over a shop, she would loudly recite, for all to hear, exactly what was written there. She was just like a kindergarten child, immensely proud of their newly acquired ability to put sounds together and form meaningful articulation. She was reading everything she possibly could. Perhaps in defiance of her brain's reluctance to cooperate in other areas, it was as if she was showing off the one skill she wanted the world to know she still possessed. She hadn't lost everything. Not yet. I could tell she felt clever when she did this, and I loved that.

When Mum had first entered full-time care, she had come armed with half a dozen crossword books folded neatly in her handbag. Recognising every crossword-lover's constant quest for a pen that works, I had loaded her up with a jumbo pack of ballpoints ready for the task. Crosswords would be her solace. If she felt alone, if she felt down, if she felt bored, she could always exercise her grey matter by solving a few clues. At that stage, we had no idea how rapid her decline would be. For a while I would catch Mum still trying to attack a crossword, but when I'd arrive she'd hastily pack the book away. It was unheard of for my mother ever to leave a crossword unsolved. Eventually she seemed to lose interest altogether. Though it seems so trivial now, my heart sank when I opened her latest puzzle book to see letters randomly scrawled all over the place, making no sense and not forming any real words at all, Mum's beautifully neat handwriting now almost illegible.

As communication with Mum grew increasingly difficult, I began to write more notes to her. She seemed to respond well at first. I'd glean a nod of comprehension where my spoken words had drawn a blank for the previous half an hour. They'd just be simple words, like 'We are going to have lunch now', 'You look lovely today' or 'Are you tired?' One day, I wrote 'I love you so much, Mum' on a little note and showed it to her. Reading it, she smiled, squeezed my hand and then gestured that she'd like the pen and paper. Surprised but excited, I handed her the pen and pad. She took considerable time and effort to jot something down for me in reply.

Again, my heart sank when she handed it back to me. Though she had begun to write 'Hi, I love you very ...', the rest of the page was covered with nothing but a series of wavy lines. What looked like 'get the box' also seemed to be written there. Was she trying to ask me for something? Get the box? What did it mean?

I was touched that she could still tell me she loved me, but no matter how much I harassed her for the rest of the cryptic note's meaning, it was a riddle I was never going to solve. Showing it to her to gain insight, I was amazed to see that what she'd scrawled on the page didn't even raise an eyebrow for her. She saw her scribble as reasonable and legible writing. My eyebrows, on the other hand, were sky high.

On Mum's seventy-fifth birthday, our family and Ben's family with all seven of Mum's grandchildren in tow visited, bearing gifts, hoping to help Mum celebrate her three-quarters of a century. Sadly, she was completely unaware of the occasion, let alone that she was indeed the birthday girl. Leafy Lodge had remembered Mum's special day, commemorating it with a big, jolly sign on the wall that read 'Happy Birthday Jeannie'. Presumably it had been there all day, but little did Mum realise.

Handing over a present and card, I was shocked when Mum began to 'read' aloud what was written on the card. She repeated the same phrases over and over and despite adopting the correct card-reading tone, she was spouting absolute gobbledygook. There were vowels and consonants coming out, but no intelligible words. Interestingly, when she came to our names at the end of the card, she managed to read them all correctly, even if she did stumble several times, repeating the same names again and again.

It was confronting to see how the simple task of reading a card was no longer simple for Mum, but probably even more alarming was the fact that she was totally oblivious to her own inabilities.

SUPERHERO DRESSING

As I have mentioned, Mum was incredibly underweight immediately prior to her admission to full-time care. Months of forgetting to feed herself had resulted in a tiny, frail frame. She weighed less than fifty kilograms and had slipped down to a mere size eight for her dresses. She looked unhealthily skinny; she didn't even look like Mum.

Once ensconced in Leafy Lodge though, indulging in three hearty meals a day plus morning and afternoon teas, she began to fill out and once again took on her familiar frame. While it was great to see Mum looking more physically robust and healthy, it was problematic where her wardrobe was concerned. I would regularly receive a friendly call to ask whether I might be able to please take Mum shopping and invest in some roomier outfits for her expanding waistline. No problem. It sounds easy in theory, right? In practice, it was anything but.

We trudged down to the local shopping centre and into one of

Mum's favourite shops. Holding up outfits, I would ask, 'Do you like this, Mum?', to which she'd beam back at me and say, 'Yes! It's lovely!' Great. Progress. By the time we worked our way to the change rooms, I had an armful of potentials for her to try.

'Okay, Mum. Let's get you in here and try these things on.'

'What do you mean? I'm not trying anything on! You try them!'

'No, Mum, we're here to get you some new clothes. You need to get undressed.'

'I will do nothing of the sort.'

'Come on, Mum.'

'You come on. I'm not getting undressed.'

It was a Mexican stand-off. With her handbag on her shoulder, she had her arms so tightly folded her knuckles were turning white. My frustration levels were rising; if I'd been in a cartoon, it would have been time for the train whistle to sound and for steam to shoot out of my ears. As I tried to wrangle her bag off her and force an arm through the armhole of a pretty floral number, we somewhat aroused the interest of the wary shopkeeper. We were virtually wrestling. Mum's cries of protest, coupled with my dogged determination to get her into something, anything, even if it was over her own clothes, were sparking some concern, not only from the staff but also among our fellow shoppers. It wasn't good.

Reluctantly, I had to back down and admit defeat. Whispering for fear of Mum's dementia-fuelled wrath, I explained my predicament and Mum's condition to the perplexed shop assistant.

She looked relieved. I took a gamble with the sizes and went with Mum to pay the bill. Mum, with a wallet bereft of all but an expired Medicare card, insisted on paying for 'my' things. Before I'd had a chance to say, 'I don't think this shop accepts American Express ... or ... um ... Medicare ...' the beautiful shop assistant had taken Mum's Medicare card, pretended to swipe it through her machine and handed a voucher to Mum to sign. She winked at me and I slipped her my credit card across the counter. I could tell it meant so much to Mum to do something 'normal' for a change. That woman's kindness was such a gift that day.

Unfortunately, this was not an isolated incident. As Mum scaled up through the dress sizes (apparently her medication also caused weight gain), I was called upon to undertake more of these fun-filled shopping expeditions. The call I dreaded the most, however, was the one to say Mum needed new bras.

Like one of life's most intriguing unsolved mysteries, where on earth all the socks go, so too were Mum's bras mysteriously disappearing, seemingly vanishing into the ether. I'd buy her new ones and then a couple of weeks later be called upon again to escort my mother to the lingerie section of our local department store for more supplies. If Mum was disagreeable when it came to trying on clothes, she was even more cantankerous when it came to over-the-shoulder-boulder-holders (as she used to fondly refer to them). Throwing a tantrum that would make a belligerent three-year-old proud, she would dig in her heels and refuse to disrobe.

A long process of bribery and enticement would follow in the stuffy, cramped change room until she'd eventually cooperate and agree to try a couple of bras on.

During those bra fittings, I also learnt (the hard way) the necessity of carrying a can of emergency deodorant with me at all times. Daily tasks that are reflex actions for us, things we remember by rote, like brushing our teeth and spraying deodorant, are nigh impossible to remember for someone suffering from dementia.

Early on in Mum's stay at Leafy Lodge, I was hanging clothes in her wardrobe when a staff member began chatting to me about what lay ahead for Mum. She told me that eventually Mum would forget the order in which to put on her clothes. She went on to say that dementia patients might put their shirt on, followed by their bra or singlet over the top. It was common for pants to be pulled on, only to be followed by an outer layer of underpants for good measure. Superhero dressing! At the time, I had my doubts, thinking surely that would never happen to Mum. It was both daunting and hard to comprehend what might lie ahead.

Years on from that discussion, I learnt that the staff member had been right. Mum needed assistance to shower, brush her teeth, do her hair and, of course, to dress. Privately, I would have loved for those dear residents to be left to their own devices just for one day. I'd provide the capes!

DIGNITY BY THE WAYSIDE

Realistically, there are certain things that have to give when you are under someone else's care and residing in an institution. There is a certain loss of dignity experienced when needing to be showered or have your undies pulled up over your nether regions by someone you don't really know (or don't remember you know). As dementia renders you unable to look after your own needs, you are forced to rely on others to perform these normally private duties for you.

My mum earnt herself quite a reputation among the Leafy Lodge staff for being less than cooperative when it came to matters of grooming and dressing. (It wasn't just me after all.) But in my eyes, she was clinging tentatively to the little dignity she still possessed. Having to submit to being showered or dressed would be humiliating for anyone; in that twilight between being fully cognisant and losing all sense of what's going on, still comprehending that you can no longer look after your own basic needs, it must be incredibly humbling to have to surrender control.

Mum had always taken pride in her appearance and was fussy about how her hair looked. She would lament over any flat spots and promptly pouf them out with a bit of teasing. She'd never leave home without her 'face on' (which used to baffle me as a kid – didn't she already have her face on? I was worried one day I'd find her with her face *off*). She had a flair for choosing styles that flattered her figure – never in contention for Trinny and Susannah's *What Not to Wear* – and could colour coordinate and accessorise with the best of them. At the same time, she was often critical of the way she looked and masked her low self-esteem with self-deprecating humour.

As a new resident of Leafy Lodge, Mum was still in control of how she dressed. She'd always wear her lippy and her flashy earrings, though Lord knows how she was able to keep track of them. I took her to get her hair cut and blow-dried a few times. The first time we went, we got her usual colour put in. Her hair was trimmed and blow-dried and looked fabulous. Not a flat spot in sight.

The next time we went, however, Mum was adamant she didn't want any colour whatsoever, stating she never had colour and didn't know what the hairdresser and I were prattling on about. After failing to convince her otherwise, the hairdresser obediently left Mum's hair to radiate its natural glory. After it was blow-dried, Mum was presented with a completely new image of herself in the mirror. She gasped, clasped her hand over her mouth in horror and stared incredulously at the white-haired woman that greeted her.

'It's white!' she exclaimed. 'Oh, my heavens!'

We had to remind her it was she who had refused the colour.

There was a resident hairdresser at Mum's facility, but I'd assumed we would be consulted regarding whether or not Mum was in need of a trim before they went ahead and took the liberty of giving her a haircut. This was apparently not the case. I was taken aback one day to see Mum had been given a most unflattering short back and sides. It had been smarmed down flat on her head and her usual puff had been snuffed. This would have been her biggest nightmare.

I don't mean to sound trivial. There's a lot more to a woman than the state of her hair and, let's face it, it's not really that important in the scheme of things. As I've always taught my kids, 'People look at the outward appearance, but God looks at the heart.'[2] However, I knew the real Jeannie would've hated this haircut. I hated it for her. I felt like she'd been violated, and I was indignant on her behalf.

I took her to her room and tried to give it a bit of a *zhoosh*, feeling overwhelmed to the point of being on the brink of tears. Didn't these people, to whom we had entrusted our precious Jeannie's care, know that she hated flat hair? How could they be so ignorant of who she was? Why did I care so much?

It came down to dignity.

If I was taking Mum out, I'd put some lipstick on for her. If the staff had dressed her in a tight, unflattering outfit, I'd gently take her up to her room and help her change into a better one. If she had a spiralling chin hair (or two), I'd pluck it out. It may sound ridiculous, but I wanted her to maintain a sense of who she was. If she were unaffected by dementia, she'd have been embarrassed by this haircut. I wanted Mum to be comfortable and I wanted her to be herself.

MALFUNCTIONING MOMENTS

For the most part, people with healthy brains take our everyday, garden variety functions for granted. One foot moves in front of the other with virtually no conscious thought. We dance, jump, run, skip and hop with relative ease, balancing all the while, flitting from one thing to another automatically. These mighty cerebral organs, housed so neatly within our craniums, so complex and wonderfully designed – still not completely understood by modern medicine – generally go about their daily duties on autopilot, without a hitch.

Dementia puts a spanner in the works. It *is* the spanner. As the brain begins to waste away, even the most menial tasks can become a struggle.

One such task for Mum was her ability to push off with one leg to propel herself upwards into my car. Admittedly, the size of my tribe dictates that I need to drive a bigger than average vehicle, so it is a slightly higher hike up into the passenger seat of my seven seater than it would ordinarily be. With one leg planted securely on *terra firma*, the other foot resting on the threshold of the passenger side and a hand holding tightly to the handle on the roof, Mum needed only to transfer her weight onto the foot in the car to launch herself up into the seat, using her hand to pull herself up if necessary. Most of us perform this motion every day without even thinking about it, but Mum was completely incapable of moving, frozen to the spot. It was as if she'd forgotten how to do it.

This happened regularly. I would stand behind her, a coach urging her on. I'd dig my shoulder in and try, unsuccessfully, to summon enough brute force to propel her into her seat, all the while shouting words of encouragement: 'Come on, Mum! You can do it! Up you go! Push yourself in, come on, Mum!'

It was no use.

She just muttered, 'I can't do this. I can't get in. I can't do it.'

She was profoundly correct. On several occasions, my mission to get her into the car and subsequently to the coffee shop simply had to be aborted. When she finally did make it into the car, one cheek on the seat and the other still hovering precariously over the doorway, it was a big job to get her to shuffle into position so I could pull the seatbelt on. I felt like I'd run a marathon in Ugg boots by the time we eventually pulled away from the curb. I needed a Plan B.

The following week, escorting Mum to the car to give it the old college try once again, I had a brainwave. I regularly volunteer to teach a couple of classes a week at our local primary school and there was a rectangular plastic basket in my car that I used to carry things to class. I could empty it, turn it upside down and Bob's your uncle – I'd have a ready-made step! It was just the right height too. Mum could put one foot in front of the other, no launching required. It worked brilliantly. Mum mounted the step with ease. All was well.

For a few weeks, that is, until the fateful day when I watched Mum tread confidently onto her plastic platform, only to hear a cracking noise as it buckled under her weight; her foot plunged through it and onto the ground. It was a shock for both of us! The basket rode up to knee level and was wedged on tight.

As awful as it was, the sight of my poor mum with a bright green plastic basket halfway up her leg gave me the giggles. I began to laugh hysterically, much to Mum's dismay. The jagged edges of the basket around the crack were sharp and even the slightest attempt at manoeuvring it down her leg elicited gasps of pain. I felt heartless, but I could not stop laughing. Eventually I managed to get her leg free, but we decided a trip to the cafe was out of the question that day. It had been quite a traumatic afternoon.

Certain there must be an easier way to help Mum into my car, I headed to the hardware store. Surely I'd be able to buy some sort of a step there? Explaining what I was after, the helpful staff member directed my attention to a plastic stepladder with wide treads and handles on the sides. This would be perfect.

The next time I saw Mum, I pulled out my new purchase from the boot of the car and encouraged her to begin her ascent. Disappointingly, the steps didn't line up too well with the car, the top step hovering well above the floor. Mum went up on both feet and balanced on the top step of the ladder, which looked a heck of a lot higher now she was teetering on it. She was breathing heavily and seemed genuinely distressed by the whole ordeal. I had to coax her down and into the car like I was talking someone down from a ledge. She was still panting and visibly anxious. What had I done? I feared she'd have a heart attack right there and then and I vowed I'd never make her ascend to those lofty heights again. The ladder was relegated to the garage and assigned to much less noble tasks, like changing light bulbs and reaching old hats at the back of the wardrobe.

An alternative way to reach that elusive passenger seat occurred to me later: perhaps we could use the small step stool I'd bought in the supermarket to help me reach my wall-mounted tumble-dryer. Why hadn't I thought of that before? It worked a treat and, for the time being at least, brought an end to the angst that had plagued our outings.

MEMORIES, MUSIC AND MANILOW

There has been much research[3] done on the benefits of music and music therapy for dementia sufferers. It is widely accepted that listening to music can have wonderful outcomes, including triggering memories. Music has the magical power to transport us back in time, to take us back to the place we were when we first heard a song. It brings to mind the people we were with and the stage we were at in our lives. Music evokes powerful emotions in us, often bringing joy and elation, reminding us of loved ones. For a dementia sufferer, music can break through memory roadblocks. It can reach beyond the disease and into the heart of the person. It can help the person we've lost to resurface, even if ever so briefly. It can also manage stress, agitation and anxiety. Dementia patients who are wheelchair bound and unable to speak have been observed to respond dramatically to the music they know and love, springing out of their chairs to dance and sing.

Our parents were always music lovers. For Ben and me, music

played a prominent part in our upbringing. All four of us shared a love of a good back beat and it was commonplace for one of us to burst through the front door with a new favourite song to introduce to the clan. We'd throw it on the turntable and give it a whirl. More often than not, we'd all fall in love with the new audio offering and we'd celebrate by having a dance together in the lounge room, Dad re-enacting the stomp moves from his heyday in the sixties, when he'd held the coveted title of 'Stomp Champion' at the Canopus Room in Manly's Hotel Pacific.

Mum and Dad shared similar tastes in music. Sunday nights were a highlight, when we'd all snuggle up on the lounge, gathered around the TV to watch *Countdown*. We loved our Aussie rock. AC/DC always got us going, as did the Sunnyboys, Dragon and Australian Crawl. Mum had a soft spot for Daryl Braithwaite, especially when he sang, 'Ooh yeah', and she adored Swanee, Air Supply, Noiseworks and Mondo Rock. She loved nothing more than a good crescendo.

My parents also shared a love for Billy Joel, Neil Diamond, James Taylor, Cat Stevens, John Cougar Mellencamp and Elton John, among others, but they branched out from one another in different musical directions too. Dad leant towards country music, while Mum had a soft spot for crooners like Edith Piaf, Frank Sinatra, Neil Sedaka and Barry Manilow.

Of all the tunes Mum enjoyed, there was no doubt that anything Barry sang would rank highly on her personal charts.

He was in a class of his own, as far as Mum was concerned. She loved Barry like Augustus Gloop loved chocolate cake. Mum and I once went to see him in concert and Mum was in heaven. Whenever Barry Manilow was gracing our turntable or cranking on the cassette deck, she'd yell, 'Turn it up!' 'Mandy' was a particular favourite; it was rare for Mum to get through a rousing rendition of that beautiful song without a tear.

Leafy Lodge always had music playing. Sometimes it was classical, sometimes it was hymns and sometimes it was old show tunes and classics, like 'Show Me the Way to Go Home', 'It's a Long Way to Tipperary' or 'My Way'. To my amusement, I once walked in to hear Rod Stewart, in his unmistakable gravelly tones, sweet-talking his audience – who seemed entirely unmoved and weren't inclined to let him know if they indeed thought he was sexy.

Many of the residents responded positively to their daily dose of audio stimulation (with the exception of Rockin' Rod), a particular tune pressing an obvious nerve and jolting them back in time. But I was yet to see Mum respond in such a way, so whenever I had her in the car with me (an achievement, as we've discussed), I was keen to play her favourite songs to see what would happen. Could they really transport her back? Would she know them? Could she still sing along? Would she still love them? Would these songs, once so precious to her, help to restore her memory? I wanted to know if the research was fair dinkum.

I made a playlist on my iPod titled 'Mum's Memories' and had it queued for when we headed out. I hit 'Play', cranked it up and waited with bated breath. Barry's soft piano intro fired up and he began to sing.

Mum's face lit up. Her eyes sparkled as she grinned from ear to ear.

'Do you know this song, Mum? Do you remember it?' I asked her. 'It's Barry Manilow – your favourite! It's "Mandy"!'

I was singing at the top of my lungs and Mum kept repeating, 'Oh, this is good stuff! This is good stuff! This is good!'

She wouldn't stop smiling! I was beyond happy. Tears of joy ran down my face as I belted out the chorus.

She seemed quite lucid. It was amazing. We were finally able to converse with relative ease in a non-stressed, non-awkward way. I wondered what was going through her mind. Where was she? Good old Barry! It had certainly hit the spot.

The wonderful Australian writer, Helen Garner, writes of her own mother, whom she is able to meet again in the music she'd loved.[4] This struck a chord with me. While Garner and her mother were in fabulous forests of Romantic piano concertos, my mother and I were at the Copa, Copacabana, spinning a pineapple-laden swizzle stick in a cocktail while we chatted to Lola and the handsome Tony, as the song goes. That day was such a special one.

* * *

After that high point, my car karaoke 'music therapy' sessions with Mum became a bit hit and miss. One other time she was bopping in her seat and head-banging as she attentively leant her ear to AC/DC's 'Long Way to the Top', her face plastered with pure joy (as was mine, in response). ButI played her 'Mandy' again and she didn't even bat an eyelid. From my limited experience, it seemed that conditions had to be just right for everything to click. Mum needed to be relaxed (which was rare), not distracted (even less likely) and in a good mood (seldom the case). If she was showing even the slightest hint of agitation or stress, her mind was consumed, and she was unable to give attention to or concentrate on anything else. Just like the early Hubble Telescope, she found it extremely hard to focus. So strange for someone who was once such a talented multi-tasker.

It was just so sad when songs I knew she'd adored left her cold. One such song was Swanee's 'Lady What's Your Name?'. Mum loved that song. Remember how I said she loved a good crescendo? This song not only has a stellar crescendo, it also features a Mum-pleasing key change. As far as Mum's tastes go, it has it all.

As the song began to whisper gently through my car speakers and I started to sing aloud, Mum's blank expression betrayed not even an iota of recognition for the song she had felt so much passion for in the past. Tears streamed down my face as the realisation dawned on me. It was as if she could hear nothing.

If you've ever done one of those jigsaw puzzles with hundreds of tiny pieces, you will know how frustrating it is when you are nearing completion and realise there are a few pieces missing. All that work and it will never be finished. You can see the finished masterpiece on the side of the box, but your puzzle still has gaping holes in it. A life with dementia feels like this in reverse. You start with a beautiful picture and can see clearly who the person is. They look just like they should, the image on the box a perfect replica of what is set before you. But gradually, pieces of the puzzle are removed, tiny piece by tiny piece, until you are left with gaping holes. This wretched disease claws at the very soul, dismantling the picture and making it almost impossible to see the essence of the afflicted person. All you are left with are lots of tiny pieces of blue that could be either sky or ocean. The picture can never be put back together again.

FADE IN, FADE OUT

Mum's disease progressed quite rapidly from her initial diagnosis. It didn't stay stagnant but seemed to go through various phases throughout its duration. Every now and then there was a shift in behaviour, sometimes subtle and other times pronounced, and a new phase was ushered in. Just when we thought we were getting used to managing her demeanour, things would take an unexpected turn and we would be forced to learn a whole new set of ways to cope with the new behaviour.

At first, as I've already noted, Mum's dementia was marked chiefly by aggression. She was angry about what was happening to her. Feisty and belligerent, she wasn't happy and we all knew it. Out of the blue, this aggression gave way to a real sadness. Mum would become weepy every time I visited. Anger underwent a dark transformation into depression and helplessness.

While her outbursts had been hard to take, it was even more distressing seeing Mum like this. She'd say awful things about wanting to end her life and talk, in graphic detail, about specific ways she would do it. I couldn't bear it. She would hold my hand and cry when I told her I had to go, and I'd feel dreadful about leaving. Tearfully, she told me she couldn't survive without her family there and couldn't live like this anymore. I alerted the staff about what Mum was threatening to do and they vowed to keep a close eye on her.

Every now and then during this time, Mum would have a rare moment of lucidity. I felt like mission control finally making contact with my astronauts after hearing nothing for days, fearing they were spinning off into outer space, never to return. 'Hello, Mum, come in! Are you there? Do you read me?' Finally, there was a crackle from the radio. Time was short. I had to make the most of the opportunity and try to reach her. It felt like we could lose contact at any moment.

'What's happening to me, Sarah? I just don't feel right. I'm not myself. Something is wrong with me. I'm not okay. I feel like my whole life is disappearing out of my head.' She looked me deeply in the eyes.

'Oh, Mum, you are not yourself. You have dementia but we are looking after you. It must be so confusing for you. Don't worry! We won't let anything happen to you. We love you very, very much.' I spurted it out as if I were a spy in the throes of death's grip, giving out the secret code to disarm the bomb that was set to explode in ten, nine, eight, seven ...

And then she was gone again. Roger that. Over and out.

Despite their brevity, and the despair Mum was feeling, these rare moments of lucidity felt like such a bonus. I'm grateful to God for these glimpses into Mum's mind.

Soon, the teary stage had more or less run its course, though Mum still had occasional episodes of crying. Enter: the Vague Stage.

AUNT CLARA

I know I'm showing my age, but one of my favourite TV shows as a child was *Bewitched*. No matter where I was at 6 pm, whether tackling my 'Maths Mentals', swimming in the pool, passing a footy with Ben or humming tunes from *Xanadu* as I rollerskated on the driveway, I'd race to get a spot on the lounge as soon as that familiar theme music chimed. I loved the fantasy of it all. Samantha Stephens could twitch that cute little nose of hers and accomplish anything. (Though having watched it since then, I must say the glamorous Mrs Stephens didn't do a lot to further the feminist cause by greeting Darrin every night on his return from work with his slippers and a drink she'd 'fixed' him in their home bar, to ease the pain of his hard day at the office ... But that's another story.)

Samantha had a lovable aunt, Clara, who could aptly be described as dithery or bumbling. Aunt Clara was no longer the spritely sorceress she'd once been and had begun to forget things. Failing to recall the spells of her youth, she was plagued by incorrect incantations and bibbidi-bobbidi-blunders, mumbling to herself incoherently all the while. Though I didn't understand at the time, Aunt Clara was a picture of someone suffering from dementia. She was the doddering old aunt who wasn't quite there anymore.

As Mum moved into this new mumbling, stuttering, incoherent stage, I knew she reminded me of someone but I just couldn't quite pinpoint who it was. Then one day, it dawned on me in an explosion of clarity (or should I say 'Clara-ty'?): Mum was Aunt Clara. She would mutter under her breath, befuddled, shuffling around, staring into space, her features configured in a faraway expression. She was so like her!

Mum still insisted on carrying her handbag with her at all times. As they used to say in that famous ad campaign of the 1970s, you can tell a lot about a woman by what's in her Glomesh bag. Well, it may not have been a Glomesh, but its contents did contain tell-tale signs of Mum's state of mind. Nestled among the plethora of tissue packets was her entire lipstick collection, most of which had lost their lids. There were also various mascara brushes, eyebrow pencils and other make-up bits and pieces she hadn't used in years. The one-hundred pack of biros that I had armed Mum with on her move into care had been cracked open and at least ninety-seven of them had found their resting place in her favourite tote. There was an odd collection of pictures Mum had torn out of magazines – not your usual recipes or handy hints, but seemingly random clippings, and so many of them. A sock, a bra, all the jewellery Mum owned and some unwrapped chocolates were kicking around in the debris. There was also, of course, her empty wallet and Medicare card, which she was still convinced was a credit card. Her bag was bulging.

Mum would clutch it so tightly to her side that the veins in her neck would pulsate. On the rare occasion she ever misplaced it, there may as well have been an air-raid siren: it was like a nuclear-level state of emergency, all systems go until that bag was unearthed. The Leafy Lodge staff had intuition that was second to none and often had an inkling as to which of Mum's neighbours had borrowed/pilfered her bag. They would spring into action and uncover the culprit in no time. Sheer relief would wash over Mum's face when, boomerang-like, her precious handbag was returned to her arm.

In the Vague Stage, it became increasingly difficult to take Mum out. 'Come on, Mum!' I'd say. 'Let's go and grab some lunch at the cafe. Do you want to come?'

She would nod in assent and smile at me but wouldn't budge even slightly from her chair.

One of the sweet Leafy Lodge staff members came up with an ingenious plan. Grabbing Mum's beloved handbag out from her clutches in one swift manoeuvre, he would then take a couple of steps backwards and teasingly wiggle it before her like a carrot before a donkey, luring her out of the comfort of her chair one anxious step at a time. Before she knew it, with she was on her feet and in hot pursuit of that precious possession, with which she was rightfully rewarded once she'd extricated herself from her roost.

* * *

Mum's language continued to decline until it became common for every sentence to get stuck in a loop. She would say, 'What's that over there-there-there-there-there-there-there-there-there-there-there-there-there-there-there-there …?'

Again, it was incomprehensible to me that Mum seemed blissfully oblivious to this incessant repetition. It took me back to the days when the record player would get stuck on a scratch and repeat itself silly. We would yell out, 'The record's stuck!' and someone would have to lift the needle up past the offending scratch and place it back on smoother grooves. If only it was as easy as resetting the needle with Mum.

One fairly good day, we were at a cafe having a bite to eat when Mum got stuck in one such loop. I looked her in the eye and said, 'Mum, do you know you just said the same sound about twenty times?' Strongly resisting the urge to break into Russell Morris's 'The Real Thing', I told Mum she had said, 'Ma-Ma-Ma-Ma-Ma-Ma-Ma-Ma-Ma-Ma-Ma-Ma-Ma-Ma-Ma-Ma-Ma-Ma-Ma-Ma-Ma-Ma- …'

'No, I didn't!'

'Yes, you did!'

She had absolutely no idea. We looked at one another and laughed.

STRUGGLING WITH THE BASICS

Sliding back the wardrobe door in Mum's room one day, I was shocked to find a bumper pack of adult nappies sitting on the shelf. I was horrified for Mum; I felt like this was something the staff should have talked over with us. When had this transition from being able to take care of the basic disposal of her own bodily waste to having to wear a nappy occurred? This was a big deal. Why hadn't we been informed?

The fact that my mum could still shower and toilet herself, when many of the other residents could not, was something of a badge of honour to me. While her brain was certainly on a downward trajectory, gradually wasting away, still having the independence to wash herself and care for her own body signified all was not completely lost. Nappies were a huge, sad step away from that.

Toilet training my own four children had been, without a doubt, one of my least favourite parental duties, only narrowly nudged out of top position by any clean-up job involving vomit.

137

Embarking on a day out with the kids sans nappies required military precision in preparation and planning. Multiple changes of clothes and towels were needed, and that was just for me. You never knew when you'd hear those dreaded words uttered: 'Mum, I need to go NOW!' It was imperative not to wander too far off the beaten track and to know where the closest ablutions block was at all times. Inevitably, accidents did happen.

When faced with one such accident in the confines of Mum's tiny bathroom, I held my breath and tried to clean up a little before having to call in reinforcements. Mum watched on, completely detached and curiously unphased by the monumental stench.

For a while, I'd suspected Mum had lost her sense of smell. I'd asked her on several occasions whether she could smell particular odours – freshly baked bread, perfume, coffee, flowers – and she'd remarked every time that she could not. I'd thrust things under her schnoz and ask, 'What do you think?' She'd give me a look that suggested she was pretending to know what it smelt like. She couldn't fool me.

Other times, like when trying on the bras, her body odour had been totally overpowering, yet when I'd lifted her blouse to her nose for evaluation, she'd just shrugged and said she smelt nothing. Not a thing! I was almost keeling over.

This bathroom incident only further cemented for me the fact that her proboscis was problematic and was most definitely not functioning as it should have been. I have since read that smell is often the first sense to disappear in the event of any cognitive impairment, and new research[5] has shown that it may in fact be an early warning sign of the onset of dementia.

* * *

Showering also became a job Mum could no longer cope with alone. She was as resistant as ever when it came to a good all-over scrub, but now it was physically beyond her as well. She was unable to wash her hair, brush her teeth or tend to any of her own personal hygiene needs. Once again, I must state that I am immeasurably grateful to the staff members who dedicate their lives to the care of our elderly parents and loved ones. They are selfless beyond belief and display compassion and devotion in all they do, with the patience of Job. It takes a very special person to work with sufferers of dementia and Leafy Lodge is fortunate to have many such saints on its payroll.

Once when I was trying to extricate Mum from her chair, a gorgeous carer informed me that Jeannie wasn't having a good day. Apparently, she'd been particularly obstinate, starting with not wanting to get out of bed that morning and then refusing to be showered. She had lashed out at the nurse, scratching him and digging her fingernails into his forearm. He rolled up his sleeve to reveal Exhibit A and I was filled with shame. But he had in no way shown me to gain sympathy or even garner an apology; rather, it was to point out the nature of Mum's current mood. In fact, he shrugged it off when I began to spew forth apologies, dismissing it as part and parcel of his profession. What a guy!

It brought back memories of having a toddler who, despite constant education from his dad and me to 'love others, never hurt anyone, share your toys and be gentle', would have a crack at anyone who looked sideways at him. I'll never forget the shame that came with collecting him from creche and noticing one or more children in tears in the obvious aftermath of a rampage. What has he done now? I'd wonder. (I should add, for the record, that this toddler has grown into a very loving, gentle and beautiful man; he is an exceptional human being, a true gentleman and very good at sharing his toys.) Walking into Leafy Lodge gave me a similar feeling, as I wondered what antics and misdemeanours my mother had been up to that week. Sometimes I was too scared to ask.

BACK ON THE HOME FRONT

From the outset of Mum's dementia, there were rumblings of a gradual shift in my parents' marriage. Now, seismic activity of Vesuvius proportions was registering on the Richter scale. Long-held roles were being reversed as the job descriptions Mum and Dad had signed up for back in 1965 were updated and reworked.

By the time their fiftieth wedding anniversary rolled around, things had drastically shifted between them. For a start, Mum wasn't even conscious of the fact they were celebrating such a milestone in their marriage. We gathered as a family, along with the handful of friends they hadn't yet isolated themselves from (or vice versa), to celebrate the momentous occasion at a local restaurant. Mum was oblivious as to why we were there. Ben had collected precious photos capturing tons of Somerville family memories, including Mum and Dad at their wedding, and he'd made a beautiful photo book for them as a present. Mum zealously flicked through it and pored over its pages throughout the day, but while the pictures brought a smile to her face, she seemed unaware of its significance.

As my mother gradually let go of her responsibilities and slipped out of her traditionally held duties within the marriage, Dad began to take the reins. This huge step didn't come easily for him.

Born in 1939 and 1941 respectively, my father and mother missed out on baby boomer status by a whisker. Despite our world's seeming obsession with pigeon-holing us all into generational groups, defining our behaviour by the decade we entered life, Mum and Dad's pre-boomer generation doesn't seem to feature that heavily in the popular press. I must admit, I wasn't even sure if their generation had a name until Google informed me they fitted squarely within the aptly named 'Silent Generation', a term coined in a 1951 *Time Magazine* article.

At the risk of generalising, many in my parents' generation hold much more traditional values than their baby boomer counterparts. My parents adhered strongly to this stereotype, with well-defined, gender-based roles within their marriage. Things were different in the sixties.

I arrived on the scene four weeks sooner than expected, early one Thursday evening in the summer of 69. (A bit young for my first real six-string, but those were the best days of my life.) Legend has it that Mum called Dad to announce my safe arrival, albeit a little prematurely, and although he was over the moon to be the father of a bonny baby girl, he decided he'd pop to the pub for a celebratory libation with the lads rather than drive twenty minutes to the hospital to see us. There was no rush; he'd make his way to the maternity ward the next morning.

Times have changed, thankfully. It's almost unheard of in this day and age for a father not to be present to witness first-hand the prodigious occasion of his offspring triumphantly exiting the womb of his beloved. Armed with weeks of birthing classes, the modern dad is on board with his stopwatch at the ready to track contractions. He knows just when to encourage his partner to breathe, when and where to apply heat packs, cool packs or any kind of pack his labouring partner may desire. He's also schooled in massage and armed with an arsenal of encouraging phrases and affirmations, which he may or may not need to utter, as he is perfectly attuned to whether his partner wants to hear from him or whether she wants him to shut up and say nothing. The modern dad is an expert in nappy changing, swaddling and feeding schedules. My beautiful husband – modern man that he is – even rose in the wee hours to change nappies and bring my babies to me for feeding.

In the household I grew up in, Dad never powdered a posterior, whipped out a Wet One or came even close to negotiating a nappy. Mum did all the cooking. Mum did all the washing. Mum did all the ironing. Mum did all the cleaning, dusting, vacuuming, tidying, scrubbing, dishwashing, sweeping and, in fact, all the housework. She took care of the kids (when we were still living at home) and all the day-to-day running of the household, including the finances.

For most of our childhood, Mum was a stay-at-home mother, only returning to the workforce when Ben and I were nearing the end of our high school years. Mum had originally begun training to become a nurse (leaving on account of the Matron being a cruel and heartless taskmaster) but had mainly worked secretarial jobs before she and Dad were joined in matrimony. She was a blisteringly fast typist with outstanding customer relations skills and became a valuable and treasured team member in the accountancy offices where she worked. This return to the world of paid employment, however, didn't kick-start any sharing of household duties in our home and neither of my parents expected it would. Dad was the primary breadwinner and held up his end of the household bargain by raking up leaves, taking care of the lawns, garden and general outdoor duties, cleaning the pool, washing the cars and taking out the garbage.

To those of us born into Generation X, and to a certain extent baby boomers, this division of labour along gender lines is enough to send shivers down the spine. Nevertheless, this was how Mum and Dad operated.

With this in mind, the turmoil that followed Mum's sudden departure from the family home had been easy to predict. Dad was left like a shipwreck survivor, clinging to a piece of flotsam, bobbing helplessly in the ocean of domesticity with no land in sight. Perhaps this was one of the reasons he'd been reluctant to let Mum enter full-time care.

Dad was seriously lacking in the domestic duties department. He didn't know how to operate the dishwasher, had no clue which buttons switched on the washing machine and wasn't sure how to use the oven or even what to do with the microwave. This is nothing against Dad, just a reflection of how the household functioned.

I am proud to say that it is possible to teach an old dog new tricks. I had the pleasure of being present when Dad, at the ripe old age of seventy-five, cracked his very first egg. After a few intensive one-on-one sessions, Dad mastered the microwave, worked out the washing machine and was ironing perfect creases in his pants in no time. He can now whip himself up some mean bacon and eggs for brekky and is washing and drying his clothes like a pro. He can change sheets, mop floors and keep the place looking spick and span. He's even looking for bargains, comparing prices at the supermarket. I am truly proud of him and the way he has stepped up to the plate. I keep telling him how proud (read: 'amazed') Mum would have been if she'd known. She'd have had to see it to believe it. Truth be told, Dad is pretty chuffed with his new 'man about the house' status as well.

Not only was it a difficult adjustment in terms of missing what Mum did for him, it was also hard for Dad to get used to not having anyone else around. Long past the dreaded 'empty nest' stage, Mum and Dad were so used to one another's company that for Dad, the silence in the house on his own was hard to take.

After Mum moved into care, Dad was diligent about visiting her, even when it wasn't easy. She fluctuated from being obsessed with seeing him to calling him names and ignoring him. One day, he and I were visiting together when Mum was in an angry phase. She leant towards Dad, beckoning him close so she could whisper what we thought would be sweet nothings in his ear. Instead, she nuzzled up to him and whispered, 'I'd like to rip your balls off.' The look on Dad's face was priceless. Just as she was no longer the Mum we knew and loved, she was far from being the wife Dad had loved all those years. She was there but not there.

One of Dad's good friends from his surf club days turned up to Leafy Lodge one day to visit his wife, Barbara. The two couples had spent a copious amount of time together in their younger years and had once been close friends, though they had recently lost touch. It was so bizarre to see Barbara and Jeannie living side-by-side in the same facility, without a clue that they had once known one another so well.

Bob was able to offer moral support to Dad, and they somewhat rekindled their friendship. Bob and Barbara's situation was quite different to my parents, though. Barbara's dementia had been diagnosed ten years earlier and Bob had been caring for her at home all those years. Eventually the severity of her condition necessitated her move into full-time care.

Barbara suffered from a different type of dementia to Mum's. Hers was Lewy body disease, also known as Diffuse Lewy body disease or LBD. In a similar fashion to other forms of dementia, Lewy body disease is caused by the degeneration and eventual death of nerve cells in the brain. The name originates from the doctor, Friedrich H. Lewy, who discovered the presence of abnormal spherical structures that disrupt the brain's normal functioning. Developing inside nerve cells, these abnormal proteins are now referred to as Lewy bodies. Lewy body disease is characterised by hallucinations and sometimes tremors, not unlike those you might typically associate with Parkinson's disease.

Barbara was always 'away with the pixies', and her hallucinations seemed very real to her. She would often carry out complete conversations with herself, moving to face the opposite direction when she replied to her own questions. Depending on her particular mood, these conversations could range from friendly banter to heated arguments, complete with expletives and shouting.

Just like Forrest Gump's famous chocolate box, you never quite knew which Barbara was going to greet you as you walked through the door. Sometimes she was full of joy, grinning ear to ear like a Cheshire Cat and waving to you from across the room like a long-lost friend. Other days she was like rolling thunder, spitting angry words at anyone who glanced in her direction. It certainly kept visitors on their toes.

SHARING THE LOAD

Leafy Lodge would host family get-togethers to mark special occasions such as Christmas, Mother's Day and Father's Day. I looked forward to them because they gave us a chance to connect with the families of other dementia sufferers. Through these gatherings, I heard many stories of experiences so similar to our own. While it was a sad situation that brought us together, it was both encouraging and comforting to know that others empathised with our plight. It was good to realise that we were not alone.

One such story stands out in my memory. It was the story of Paul, who developed early onset dementia at fifty-three years old – only a few years older than Ben and I were at that time. As his wife shared his story with me through tears, I truly felt for her and her teenage kids. No age is ideal where dementia is concerned, but at fifty-three there should be so much more of life left to live. If I felt ripped off being robbed of my mother and my kids' grandmother, how must this family have felt?

Paul seemed completely unable to communicate and would display random spurts of aggression. One day he pushed Mum, which raised Dad's shackles, though it is hard to hold a dementia patient accountable for their actions when they are clearly not behaving like their normal self. Our experience at Palatial Palace had taught us that.

Paul had to wear protective headgear in the end, as he was prone to banging his head against any hard surface he could find. With his head suitably padded, he would prowl down corridors looking like a front-row forward, ready to tuck into a scrum or make a tackle at any given moment.

There was another notable couple that resided in Leafy Lodge. At any time of the day, these two could be found snuggling on the lounge together, holding hands or cuddling up to each other affectionately. PDA was not a problem for this gorgeous old pair. Everyone assumed they had entered their new accommodation as a married couple, but surprisingly this was not so. They had discovered one another upon taking up residence in Leafy Lodge and, like smitten teenagers, were besotted, each unable to be away from the other's side. Apparently this is not an uncommon occurrence in care. I couldn't help but feel for the poor man's wife, who would find her husband canoodling with another woman whenever she popped in to see him.

Many of the residents in care, the women in particular, have spent much of their lives caring for others – nurturing their children and heaping love on their spouses. So, it's understandable that when put into this new environment, they want to care for one another and attend to each other's needs. It wasn't uncommon in Leafy Lodge to see someone mothering another by making sure their serviette was correctly on their lap, wiping a milk moustache from a top lip or tucking in a wayward piece of hair. Often, I was the recipient of a stranger's warm embrace, an affectionate hand rub or a pat on the back. When my daughter Maisy, who is extremely understanding and beautifully patient with people, came with me to visit her nanna, women would come out of the woodwork to hold her face in their hands or stroke her hair, presumably reminded of what it was like to love and devote themselves to their own offspring.

Many dementia sufferers respond positively to cuddling and caring for a baby doll, and while this behaviour definitely seemed a little unusual when I first witnessed it, seeing the love in the eyes of an elderly mother as she clutched a faux baby to her breast would bring a lump to my throat every time. There was also a very loved and much patted toy dog at Leafy Lodge, life-sized and battery operated, that wagged its tail, barked intermittently and snuggled up on the residents' laps when they needed a companion. From time to time, real dogs were brought in as therapy animals. It's amazing how much comfort and calm these little furry friends bring.

A dementia facility is a place where nothing is out of the ordinary.

My wonderful friend Keryn and I were visiting Mum one day when she was listening to and observing what her fellow residents were doing across the circle from us. One of them was convinced she'd lost her train ticket and was asking everyone within a half mile radius of her imaginary train station whether they had seen it. She had to be on the six o'clock train and was sure that without her ticket, her friends would leave without her. She was distraught, going from person to person, pleading through tears for any information on the whereabouts of her ticket. The staff did an amazing job of offering their comfort and managing to console her with the assurance they'd help her locate the lost ticket and get her on that train.

Another woman was convinced she was in Leafy Lodge for a holiday and would be going home in the next few days. She said it was a good thing because the food was 'terrible'. Mum leant over to Keryn and, with a not-so-subtle circular finger motion in front of her ear, whispered behind her hand that the people in this place were a sandwich short of a picnic.

Cheryl was the resident flasher, who regularly lifted her shirt to reveal her braless 'fun-bags', as Mum would have said, for all to see, though no-one so much as raised an eyebrow. Then there was Elsie, who liked to go nude from the waist down – again, not really causing any sort of stir whatsoever. Henry loved to yodel and did his best to transform Leafy Lodge into a Swiss chalet. If you closed your eyes, you could almost hear the cow bells clanging. I have a soft spot for Henry, because every time I saw him, he'd say, 'Gee, you're a good sort!'

Joe liked to eat a meal and then change seats so he could be served another one. We all loved the fact that he didn't think anyone was onto him.

After lunch one day, Anna proceeded to eat her serviette.

I've also witnessed a stand-off between the bossy Jan and meek and mild Paul. Jan told Paul he could no longer sit with her because he was 'boring'. She told him that none of the women liked him and that he needed to sit somewhere else. Dear Paul obediently got up from the table, but decided to take all the cutlery and hold it for ransom. Not happy, Jan.

Mavis liked to collect (read: 'steal') surgical gloves from the nurse's cart and tie them in knots. She once proudly informed me she was fashioning a rope so she could make an escape. Judging by the length of this latex masterpiece, she was envisaging a Rapunzel-style drop from a lofty tower. It's a shame Leafy Lodge is only one storey high.

Greeting a new resident one day, I said, 'Hi, I'm Sarah. What's your name?' She replied, 'Nothing because I keep having to go into the club and get changed. This one's only up to my chin.'

The Leafy Lodge staff worked hard to provide stimulating activities for the residents. From cooking demonstrations to silent discos, games of charades and portrait painting – there was always something fun to do. One day, recreation officer Jennifer, Leafy

Lodge's answer to Julie from *The Love Boat*, wrote the letters of the alphabet on the whiteboard, and then asked the residents to come up with a first name for each respective letter. It was all going like clockwork – 'A for Arthur, B for Bob, C for Charlie...' When it came to 'S', like a cheeky little schoolgirl, Mum yelled out at the top of her voice, 'SEX!'

BIRTHDAY BOTCH-UP

As Mum's dementia progressed, she seemed more and more reluctant to go out – the total opposite of her sheer desperation to break out of the place when she'd first arrived. People had warned us that she would become 'institutionalised' and eventually feel at home where she was, but it had seemed like such a far-fetched notion back then. The sound of someone being institutionalised frightened me, so I had hoped there was no truth in the matter. As time passed, when I visited and suggested we steal away for a cup of tea in the real world, she seemed almost super-glued to the comfy armchair (with its protective plastic coating) and would refuse even to stand up.

When Mum's seventy-sixth birthday rolled around, we thought it would be nice if we and all the kids took her out for a slap-up lunch in the fancy cafe with the grand piano, not far from Leafy Lodge. It was a splendid idea, in theory.

Mum was over the moon to see us all, greeting us with a big grin, hands clasped with glee: Ross and I and our four kids, Ben and Julie and their son Will. We crowded around our matriarch. In her mirth and excitement, she began shooting out rapid-fire kisses into the air towards us. While she may not have been able to articulate it verbally, she made known the extent of her love for us through this extravagant gesture. It was beautiful and amused the kids no end.

We tried to explain the delicious excursion that awaited but Mum showed no inclination to shift from her roost. After a lot of coaxing, we somehow managed to extricate her from the sticky chair and lure her out through the series of Maxwell Smart-style coded doors into the broad daylight. Ben and I had parked our cars next to each other with a vacant spot in between. We decided Ben's car would be easier for Mum to get into (we've already discussed the trauma associated with getting Mum up and into my car). My nephew, Will, got into the car and began calling to his nanna, patting the seat beside him and promising more kisses if she got in.

He almost had her over the line, but at the last minute she aborted the mission. Ross then bravely tried to tempt her up onto the step stool and into the back of our car. Again, she looked keen, but then decided it was all too hard.

This vacillation went on for half an hour. We felt like we were at the tennis, eyes darting from one car to the other as her indecision persisted. We were getting nowhere. In the end, we conceded defeat, and Mum led the charge back through the many coded doors, into the comfort of the place she now called home. It was extraordinary that the very place Mum had fought to leave was now the object of her longing, the place she most desired to be. Never in my wildest dreams had I thought this would be possible. So many questions filled my head: Would she ever leave again? Was this it? Would we have to resign ourselves to the fact that Mum was never going to set foot out of this place?

Given her reluctance to leave, you can imagine my astonishment when, a little while after the birthday fiasco, Mum greeted me and, moments after laying eyes on me, scooped up her handbag and leapt out of her chair towards me with the expectant words 'Let's go!' rolling off her tongue. I'd resigned myself to the fact that there would be no more outings so this was quite a surprise, to say the least.

'Okay,' I said confidently, though I had absolutely no clue where I was going to take her. I was just buoyed along by the prospect of another car trip with Mum and the realisation that we had been wrong in our assumption she wouldn't ever leave again. Bravo! Let's go!

Surprisingly, the entry into the car was accomplished with relative ease. It was quite uneventful, in fact. We drove to a nearby club, which I knew had a nice coffee shop, and disembarked, again without a hitch. So far, so good. I then had to physically steer Mum across the road and through the doorway to get into the cafe, which was no easy task. It reminded me very much of trying to navigate an abundantly laden trolley through a full carpark at a shopping centre, the trolley hindered by that ubiquitous wonky wheel. I had the feeling that if I left her to her own devices, she'd career off into a gutter somewhere and be stuck there for days.

Eventually we arrived at the cafe and found a seat. I ordered a couple of cups of tea and was given a number to pop on the table, but it was dangerously close to closing time and the staff were preoccupied with their end of day duties. It seemed our beverages had taken a back seat to cleaning the coffee machine and wiping crumbs from the counter. Mum was extremely restless. She was a time bomb. I tried to reassure her that the tea was coming and convince her to sit tight, but I soon realised that, in actual fact, they had forgotten us.

I was in a dilemma. Do I leave Mum at the table by herself while I wander over to the counter to ascertain the whereabouts of our tea? Or, do I get Mum up and bring her with me, risking the chance that she won't sit back down again? I decided I had to bring her with me to the counter, where the staff were very apologetic, promising our tea would be served pronto. Unfortunately, it was not 'pronto' enough, as Mum was now refusing to sit down, weaving in and out of the club's tables. I gave chase, our table number wedged firmly under my arm, eventually managing to corner her and lure her to our table. By the time we made it back to our seats, our steaming cups were there waiting for us. They were piping hot – too hot to drink – and Mum decided she was adamantly opposed to drinking hers at all. Great. She bobbed up and down in her seat like a jack-in-the-box, mumbling incoherently and showing a great desire to leave. I asked for two takeaway cups to pour the tea into. In hindsight, it was a dumb idea, but I think the effort it took to get the damned tea made me feel like I'd better not leave it behind.

The cups had no lids and were burning my hands, so steering Mum back to the car was a little tougher this time around. She stopped by the side of the road and refused to move. With both my hands occupied by the searing tea, all I could do was beg her to move. She would not. I tried my best to stay calm, but Mum wasn't budging. I guzzled down the two cups of molten tea in fast succession, stripping tastebuds off my tongue left, right and centre in the process.

'Come on, Mum. Let's go back. Look, there's the car, just over there.

'Come on, Mum. We can't stay here all day.

'Let's just walk over to the car, Mum.

'Come on, Mum.

'Come. On. Mum!'

I reckon we were there for a good twenty minutes.

Arriving at the car was a major relief, but the fun and games weren't quite over. After we drove into the Leafy Lodge carpark, Mum decided she would not alight from the vehicle. She did not want to get out of that car and nothing I tried even came close to making it happen. I attempted to gently pull her out, all the while coaxing her with my 'Come on, Mums'. This was not going well.

Meanwhile, my rapid-fire tea drinking had had the adverse effect of causing my bladder to become bursting at the seams. I was busting. I appealed to Mum and implored her to get out of the car, as I was about to wet my pants. I considered leaving her there, locking her in the car, but it was a very hot day and a decent walk to the toilet. I didn't want her to overheat or panic, nor did I want to be arrested for locking an elderly woman in a boiling hot car. At least I hadn't taken her to the casino.

Pointing at some shrubbery, Mum suggested quite matter-of-factly that I 'just go in the garden'. She said it with a deadpan face, like it was the most obvious option in the world.

'How about instead,' I said through gritted teeth, 'you just get out of the flipping car so I can go to the toilet!' Please. Pretty please. Pretty please with ice cream on top.

Finally, Mum cooperated and I made it to the loo within minutes of public disgrace, my cup perilously close to having runneth over.

I'd discovered the hard way that it really wasn't possible to take Mum out anymore. The most difficult thing about that for me was the fact that I could no longer have Mum all to myself. There'd be no more one-on-one time. Forevermore, my visits with my mum would be shared with all her quirky neighbours. We'd always have to meet in that same environment. It was a blow.

THE SEASON TO BE JOLLY

Ever since I can remember, Christmas has been a really special celebration for our family. Now that I'm older, I understand the significance of Christmas being the celebration of Jesus' birth, but as I was growing up, Christmas meant mainly two things: presents from Santa and 'Grandma Potatoes'. Sure, the carols were great, we had fun putting up the Christmas tree, sitting on Santa's knee, reading corny jokes from the bonbons ... but nothing beat Grandma Potatoes. As the name suggests, my grandma, 'Pearl' Somerville, was the original mastermind behind these scrumptious, crunchy spuds. As the grandchildren paired off and married and families spread out across the city, in-laws began pulling us in different directions; it became impossible for us all to meet in one place on Christmas Day and eventually Grandma passed away. But while things have changed and Grandma is sadly no longer with us, her legendary potatoes live on – a legacy I'm sure she'd be infinitely proud of.

Mum was always at the helm on Christmas Day. It could be forty degrees Celsius outside, but Mum would be slaving over a hot stove, sweat on her brow, basting the expertly stuffed turkey, chopping pumpkin, topping and tailing the beans, stirring the homemade gravy and, of course, getting those Grandma Potatoes how Goldilocks would've liked them: just right. Many a Christmas Day lunch was delayed, ravenous Yuletide revellers salivating in anticipation, while Mum announced her characteristic apology: 'Sorry it's taking so long, we're just waiting for the potatoes!' It was always worth the wait.

Mum and Dad kept the same Christmas tree for their whole lives. I've spied it in the faded photo albums of my first Christmas. (There was also a cute little potted rubber tree-come-Christmas tree they'd made the mistake of planting in the garden a year or two later, from where it eventually took over the entire front of the house and weaselled its way into every nook and cranny of our household plumbing. Should've kept it in that little terracotta pot. Ah, if only we'd known.) The Christmas tree, which, as evidenced by the photo, was admittedly a little more luxuriant in the foliage department back in 1969, was only four-foot tall, if it was lucky. The plastic tree was more of a shrub really, covered in plastic red berries that have miraculously survived to this day and would never be allowed in this modern age of Occupational Health and Safety, Due Diligence, Choking Hazard Awareness, etcetera, etcetera.

Mum was a bit partial to those little red berries and loved the fact that our Christmas greenery was so unique. Its sparse branches were adorned with the fruits of our crafty labour over the decades – cotton-ball snowmen with toothpick arms, egg-carton angels with pipe-cleaner halos and reindeer expertly crafted from bottle lids and spray-painted sticks. As 25 December drew nearer, our special little tree would almost disappear in a sea of presents. The gold star on the top could just be seen poking its festively gleaming prongs up above the gifts.

Mum loved playing Santa. She had a knack for choosing just the right gift for everyone and genuinely preferred giving to receiving. As we got older, although I was happy to continue the fantasy, Ben was on a quest to prove Santa's fraudulent identity. He would lead me around the house, madly searching for the Christmas loot, convinced Mum and Dad were masquerading as the man in the red suit. I'd tag along as a firm sceptic, but one year my naïvety was tested. Standing on the stepladder, peering into the top shelf of Mum and Dad's wardrobe, Ben excitedly proclaimed, 'Sarah, look! I told you Santa wasn't real!'

Through my brother's enthusiastic coaxing, I allowed my own peepers to roam around the expanse. I clearly saw a Shogun Warrior, a Barbie Fashion Face and, to my delight, Stretch Armstrong himself. Wow! This was exactly what had been on our lists! Ben was triumphant but I wanted to check with Mum. Surely there had to be a good explanation.

We summoned Mum and showed her exhibits A, B and C,

still residing in their not-so-clever hiding place. In what can only be described as an Academy Award-winning performance, she exclaimed, 'What! Where did these come from? Oh, my goodness!' She was as shocked as we were. 'Stretch who? Never seen him before in my life.'

She shot a perplexed look at us, as if we were some sort of crime-solving trouble-shooters and, with a pensive scratch of her chin, came up with what I thought was a very plausible explanation: perhaps Santa, foreseeing his itinerary would be rather full on Christmas Eve, had ingeniously thought to hide the presents ahead of time? Ben wasn't buying it, but to Little Miss Gullible this seemed like a completely believable scenario. What a brilliant mother I had. Talk about thinking on your feet.

* * *

The first Christmas we realised all was not well with Mum, we had gathered in the lounge room, giving out the presents. As she was handing around the gift-wrapped goodies, it became apparent that Mum had forgotten to buy gifts for two of her grandchildren. She was apologetic but seemed to brush it off quickly, mostly unperturbed. This was not like Mum at all. She'd normally have been mortified to have had such a devastating Christmas shopping fail. The girls were very gracious and didn't even bat an eyelid, but it was a worrying sign.

When Mum entered full-time care, Christmas changed forever.

We would pick her up on Christmas morning and bring her home to be with us. Julie and Ben and Ross and I took turns to host, alternating who took on the mantle, slaving over the hot stove and perfecting those special spuds. It wasn't the same but there was a palpable joy in just having her there. She could still unwrap her presents, enjoy the atmosphere and partake in some Grandma Potatoes. With Dad home alone now, his enthusiasm for decking the halls had waned. The little Christmas tree with the red berries was never brought out of its box again.

The hardest Christmas of all was the year Mum was no longer able to come out. After the birthday debacle, it was all too difficult. As much as we toyed with the idea of bringing her home, it would have been too stressful for all of us and, most importantly, for her. We gathered at Leafy Lodge instead, descending en masse to shower our mother and nanna with gifts, hugs and kisses. After a short while, she grew very restless and anxious and seemed overwhelmed. She had been tickled pink to have us all there, but we knew it was time to go. Having to say goodbye and head back to celebrate without Mum felt cruel and unnatural. As she tearily farewelled us, not really understanding why or where we were going, we were all biting our lips to hold back our own tears.

That same year was the first time Julie's Great Nan Edna had not been able to leave her full-time care to spend Christmas with us either. The difference was that it was Edna's body that had deteriorated, not her mind. At ninety-seven, Edna was still as sharp as a tack. In fact, just a couple of years earlier I'd received a Facebook friend request from ninety-five-year-old Edna. That's not something that happens every day! In comparison, Mum was in her mid-seventies, her body in great shape but her mind an ever-shrinking mass of grey matter rattling around, echoing inside her beautiful skull.

SHORT BACK AND SIDES

It's fair to say Mum has always had a love-hate relationship with hairdressers. Within seconds of that Velcro tab on the back of the protective plastic apron being ripped open, we'd know one way or the other, whether she was a fan of the new coiffure or whether she was contemplating wearing a paper bag over her head for the foreseeable future. I mentioned earlier that she'd had a few less-than-flattering dos at the hands of the resident stylist at Leafy Lodge, but she'd been ignorant (blissfully or otherwise) as to how they'd looked. Somewhere in the recesses of Mum's mind, however, there must have been an override switch: she was able to detect a hairdresser at fifty paces. She'd begun to refuse point-blank to allow the hairdresser to cut, colour, style, brush, curl, comb or come within a centimetre of her lengthening tresses with anything even closely resembling scissors. Apparently, this had happened the three times the poor hairdresser had visited.

Dad and I had decided to see Mum on a particular day when

the aforementioned hairdresser was doing the rounds. The staff had given us the heads up (pun intended) and asked us politely if we might be able to encourage Mum to have a much-needed trim.

Predictably, Mum was vocally opposed and adamantly defiant, refusing to get out of her chair. Dad and I devised a plan whereby he would go behind the chair and tip Mum out into my waiting arms. Once she was up, we'd each take an arm and gently guide her to the hairdresser's pop-up parlour. Good in theory but not so successful in reality. Mum shrieked like a banshee, transforming herself into an MMA pro, kicking, punching and scratching Dad and me, and the long-suffering staff-member who'd leapt to our aid. Who would have thought a haircut could be so traumatic?

The look of sheer hatred on Mum's face as she set about plunging her pretty, painted talons deep into our fleshy forearms and kicking us in the shins like a spoilt schoolgirl was not only quite terrifying but also heartbreaking. Such incredibly uncharacteristic behaviour for someone normally so loving.

In nothing short of a miracle, we managed to wrangle Mum into a chair but every time the stylist would clip a specially selected little section of hair into place, Mum would swiftly reef the clip from her head and throw it across the room with an overarm Warnie would have been proud of. All the while, she continued to gush forth a tirade of abuse, directed at all of us. That saintly hairdresser worked wonders, snipping her moving target into a not-bad-at-all-considering style, conceding as she did so that my mother was indeed the most 'trying' client she'd had ... ever. A Bex and a good lie down were certainly in order after that ordeal, and not just for the hairdresser.

As we were in the throes of coercing Mum into the hairdresser's chair, one of the staff members, whom I greatly admire and respect, stared straight at me and mouthed, 'Is it really worth it?' At that stage, I felt like we'd already committed to the process and to back out would have seemed futile. I'd shrugged back and averted my eyes to the heavens. Was it worth it? That was a good question. With the benefit of hindsight, I'd definitely agree that it monumentally was not worth it. After that day, I decided I would encourage Mum to grow her hair down to her bum and to wear it in a bun. Haircuts shmaircuts. So overrated.

SLAP-STICK ALL THE WAY

With Mum's ability to communicate rapidly diminishing, it became harder and harder to visit. If conversation had previously been hard, it was now near impossible. She would plant herself in her favourite chair, stare into space and make repetitive sounds non-stop, rarely uttering a recognisable word, though her tone and gestures strongly suggested she thought she was making complete sense. Her most common combinations were centred around the 'ack' sound and the 'ang' sound; for example: 'back-back-back-mack-mack-mack-pack-pack-pack-backa-backa-macka-macka' or 'manga-manga-manga-nanga-nang-manga-manga-nang-nanga-nanga-nanga'.

At other times, an actual word would set the tone for the babble. She might point to someone's shirt that was blue and say the word 'blue' followed by 'boo-boo-bool-loo-boo-boo-blue-boo'. The babble could go for the length of a conversation, my nods and 'Oh, reallys' filling in the gaps. Mum has always been a sucker for a good fashion accessory, so if ever I came to visit wearing a colourful necklace or some big earrings, she would point to them and I would know the gist of what she was trying to say. It was a good catalyst for a chat. I'd start with, 'Oh, you like this, Mum?', to which she would nod in assent, and I'd waffle on about the colours or where it came from. Mostly, I don't think she understood my words but occasionally I'd see a spark of recognition. As time went on, those sparks became rarer.

One way I found I could communicate with Mum, or at least get her to laugh, was by pulling funny faces. Come to think of it, she always did love a good face pull (remembering, of course, that it could only be fleeting, lest the dreaded wind-change cause it to permanently fix upon your features). If I poked out my tongue, Mum would copy and we'd both have a good giggle. Before long, we were fish-facing with the best of them and my repertoire of animal impersonations was growing.

A meal-time favourite – simple but effective – was to put the serviette on my head like a hat. Grabbing the napkin, quoting from the motion picture masterpiece, *Flying High*, I would say, 'Sarah, what do you make of this? Well … I can make a hat or a brooch or a pterodactyl!' As the serviette flapped its dinosaur wings past Mum's eyes, she would laugh out loud, making my day.

A faux fall or trip or pretending to miss the chair and land on my bot-bot always raised a smile. Slap-stick became an icebreaker. At times, by the looks my antics were garnering, I'm sure the Leafy

Lodge staff members were contemplating whether they should make up a room for me.

* * *

Mum never left us in any doubt that her love for us was immense. This remained a constant, no matter how much her dementia twisted and contorted the rest of her personality. Whenever she saw me and I'd take a seat beside her, she'd tilt her head to the side, her beautiful smile bursting with love, and stroke my hand or pat my shoulder affectionately. Long after most of Mum's vocabulary had retreated, she could still utter, 'I love you' as clearly as ever. Later, when even those words struggled to come together, the smile and the head tilt would be accompanied by an 'awwww' that I knew was 'I love you'.

When she was up and about, she would take me by the hand and parade me before the staff, proudly announcing, in her own garbled way, to all and sundry, that I was her beautiful daughter. At other times, while sitting together in silence, she would stare lovingly at me before planting kisses upon my cheeks or lifting the back of my hand to her lips, forever demonstrative in her overflowing love.

If I looked deeply into her eyes, I could always see them brimming with affection. Now that I have my own kids, I know that nothing is as strong as a mother's love. My mother always has, and always would, love me fiercely.

JOINING THE GOOPS

Don't read this chapter while eating.

When I was in primary school, I learnt a poem called 'The Goops' by Gelett Burgess. It went like this:

The Goops they lick their fingers,
And the Goops they lick their knives;
They spill their broth on the tablecloth–
Oh, they lead disgusting lives!
The Goops they talk while eating,
And loud and fast they chew;
And that is why I'm glad that I
Am not a Goop – are you?

Mum loved this poem, learning it off by heart and quoting it often. We'd laugh at those dreadful Goops, quietly thankful our manners were (usually) impeccable. On the odd occasion our guard would slip and we'd deign to lick a knife or Ben would direct us to

'Look at those ceiling mouldings' to divert our attention while he hoovered the bottom of his ice cream bowl – sans spoon – Mum would question us with disgust: 'You're not joining the Goops, are you?'

With my mother now tightly held in the grip of dementia, one might have been compelled to ask her the same question. Her behaviour had become quite Goop-like indeed. The real Jeannie Somerville would have been absolutely horrified if she had witnessed how she was conducting herself in such an un-mannered manner.

On one particular day, I had timed my visit to coincide with the lunch hour so I could share a meal with Mum. We were seated together at a big oval table with a bunch of Mum's fellow residents. As the bibs were being donned, I noticed Mum attending to a small pile of unidentified morsels on the table. She was shuffling the tiny pieces back and forth, arranging them in patterns on the placemat. Before I had time to ask, 'What on earth is that?' she had reached over her shoulder to obtain another piece for the pile, which I discovered was a fragment of an odious back mole she had been gradually dismantling over the course of the morning. Ew! I watched on in disbelief as my mother, keeper of courtesy, espouser of correct etiquette, normally profoundly well-mannered, continued to pick her mole and add its disgusting pieces to her small heap, right there at the table where we were eating. I felt like throwing up.

Mum also had a great aversion to spitting, reminding us of the countless germs contained in every wayward squirt of saliva. I must admit, I am not a fan myself. Whenever I see a footballer hacking up phlegm and depositing it in globules on the field, it makes my stomach turn. I feel for the player that gets tackled and cops a face-full, sliding right into that delightful little deposit. Did you know it's illegal to spit in the streets of Singapore? You can be fined up to $1000 for public spitting. In an effort to prevent such anti-social behaviour in my own offspring, I would often tell them this fact, ignoring their 'But we don't live in Singapore, Mum!' smarty-pants retorts.

Given Mum's track record in decorum, you can imagine my horror the first time she leapt up from her chair to walk into the hallway, cough up a big mouthful of spittle and project it forcefully onto the floor ... inside, no less! With a look of satisfaction and a gentle dusting together of the hands, she returned guiltlessly to her seat, completely oblivious to the fact she had committed such a major breach of etiquette in broad daylight. I doubt even the Goops would stoop that low.

A CATASTROPHIC TURN OF EVENTS

Dad was in Queensland, holidaying for a couple of weeks, when the weather bureau forecast blistering conditions in our area for the following day, prompting police to instigate evacuations from properties that might be in the line of fire, so to speak. As luck would have it, I had come home from work a couple of hours early to try to sleep off a mind-splitting migraine. I was woken from my deep slumber by my daughter handing me the phone, saying, 'I think it's about Nanna.'

I grabbed the phone, barely compos mentis, and was informed that Leafy Lodge, along with all of its cerebrally challenged occupants, was to be evacuated due to the forecast 'Catastrophic Fire Danger'. As far as I knew, 'catastrophic' was a whole new category of fire danger. A deadly combination of soaring temperatures (thirty-seven degrees Celsius), a long dry spell and a prediction of blustering winds had raised the alarm. While terrible, out-of-control fires had been raging in the north of our state, we were yet to even have a fire in Sydney. Who ever heard of evacuating areas before there's a fire? Nevertheless, as the old adage goes, It's better to be safe than sorry (or, as the lesser-known adage goes, It's better to be evacuated than to get burnt in a bushfire). So, Leafy Lodge's frail residents were to stay with their nearest and dearest for two nights at least, until the weather had cooled and the danger subsided. I was told to be there within the hour.

This was a lot to digest. Thankfully, the Panadols I had downed an hour before had kicked in and my snooze had gone a long way towards ridding me of my pesky migraine. I called Ross and left a voicemail to let him know his mother-in-law was coming to stay, and alerted Ben of this extraordinary predicament that was being thrust upon us. It was daunting, to say the least.

Punching in the required codes, I entered Leafy Lodge to find a frenzy of activity. Bewildered residents were being ushered, arm-in-arm with their loved ones, out the doors. Bags were being packed, orders barked, names checked off lists and medications issued. It was chaos. I was eternally grateful that Molly had offered to come with me for moral support.

Mum was happy to see us, welcoming us both with an ear-to-ear grin, but she was not showing any desire whatsoever to leave the comfort of her favourite chair. No amount of verbal persuasion was going to get us over the line, so we had to pull out the big guns. Two of the staff members gave each other a knowing look that said, 'Let's just do what we have to do', before retrieving an ice-cold beer from the fridge to wave enticingly before my mother.

Her eyes lit up upon seeing the cool libation, but she wasn't to be easily fooled today. They would have to dig deep and pull out the biggest weapon in their arsenal – Mum's beloved handbag. I was amused to see it so close to hand. It seems they had it permanently stashed behind the desk, at the ready for situations just like the one we now found ourselves in. Sure enough, seeing her precious tote being temptingly brandished before her stirred an impulse to get up and follow. With gentle persuasion from one of her favourite staff members, she was up.

As Molly and I led my incredulous mum out through the series of security doors and into the bright blue of the day outside, she could hardly believe it. I think it had been about two years since she had left the facility. Accompanied by a little giggle, she darted her head from side to side, glancing from us to the door to the surroundings and back again in quick succession. With the look of a guilty little girl plastered across her face, the realisation seemed to hit her at once: she was free!

She climbed into Molly's nice, low-to-the-ground car without much ado and quietly took in the view from her window as we drove to our place. My head was swimming with instructions about medication, showering and adult nappies, and unwanted memories of the last time Mum had visited came flooding back. Could I really do this? It seemed insurmountable. I felt for those elderly spouses who were being forced to bring their mentally depleted partners home. The whole reason their loved ones had been placed in care in the first place was their sheer inability to cope with the constant demands of nursing an individual with dementia. The situation was bizarre.

In the five years since Mum had last been our house guest, her dementia had become a different beast. Irrational anger, violence and an unquenchable desire to go home had been replaced, for the most part, by a placid and laid-back attitude. An adamant belief that there was nothing whatsoever wrong had been replaced by a docile complacency; vicious words that tore at the very fabric of our beings now gave way to incessant, nonsensical jibber-jabber. Maybe it wouldn't be as bad as I was expecting.

Taking time off work, my gorgeous brother came to stay with Mum so I could fulfil my regular teaching commitments for the day. My niece Sophie brought the family's fluffy puppy Winki to visit, providing Mum with a nice diversion, once she'd warmed to him.

The day was going swimmingly. Swimmingly, that is, until it was time for Mum's medication. Getting her to swallow that tiny sliver of a half tablet was tantamount to getting her to eat a leopard's testicle. She spat that thing out like it was poison. After several failed attempts, I passed the baton to Ben, who bravely took up the cause. No amount of trickery, not even hiding it in a teaspoon of jam, was going to get that damn drug into her. She had another much bigger pill, too, which I'd attempted to squish through the impenetrable barrier of her tightly pursed lips, but to no avail. And then there was the oral medicine she had to be convinced to swill back not once, not twice, but three times a day. Ben kept at it until he was miraculously able to accomplish her ingestion of the two pills and one dose of the medicine. It had only taken six hours.

* * *

Mum seemed genuinely happy during her stay with us. She took a shine to being around while I performed mundane tasks like hanging the washing out and cooking dinner. These things had been the fabric of her existence for so many years and it had never really occurred to me that she'd miss them. It dawned on me that it had been over five years since she'd been a part of a functioning household. Mum let herself in and out of our back door and took delight in taking command of the clothesline, feeling pants' legs, flipping tea towels and turning t-shirts, assessing whether or not it was time to bring them in. Watching this simple act took me back and reminded me how much Mum had taught me. I now feel the pants' legs, flip the tea towels and turn the t-shirts just like she does. I see Mum in myself and vice versa. My movements are intrinsically hers.

As my hair greys and my skin loses its youthful glow, occasionally I glance at myself in the mirror and catch a glimpse of Mum. I have her fading eyebrows, her little feet, her freckly hands. So much of what I do and the way I do it comes from years of watching her glide through life before me. Now, we had come full circle. It was as if I was the mother and she was the child. There I was keeping an eye on her, keeping her safe, and making sure she had enough to eat.

* * *

If Mum had a slight aversion to showers before, now she detested them. I had the unenviable task of getting her clean. Taking a deep breath and mumbling a muffled prayer, I managed to get her undressed and into the bathroom, where she halted abruptly as she caught sight of all her naked glory reflected back at her in the full-length mirror. The small mirror above the sink in her bathroom at Leafy Lodge, like most mirrors, doesn't cater for the vertically challenged like Mum (or me – the apple doesn't fall far from the tree). I'm lucky if I can spy my eyebrows in Mum's mirror when I'm on tippy toes, so this panorama of pink must have been quite a sight for Mum to take in. For someone who generally wasn't fond of mirrors, Mum's fascination with her reflected image was hilarious. With a general air of admiration, she smiled at herself and fluffed her hair as she gave herself the once-over more than once over. It was refreshing to see that she liked what she saw.

It was there, however, that the hilarity left the building and the obstinate Jeannie arrived – uninvited, mind you. The shower was running at the perfect temperature and all Mum had to do was step inside. Heck, we could leave the door open if she wanted to. It sounds simple right? Well ... if only. She flatly refused to get in. My attempts at washing her down with a soothing, warm face washer – a little something I'd prepared earlier – were met with shrieks and an uppercut that missed my chin by a whisker and knocked the washer out from my grip. Copping a death stare that would terrify a small child, I decided to pull up stumps and opt for the old 'shower in a can' instead. At least she smelt good.

Next on the agenda in our nightly ritual was for Mum to don the PJs and a 'night nappy'. During the day, she was getting around in pull-up type pants, which were relatively easy to get on and off. This night nappy, however, was not so user-friendly. It was a gigantic version of a baby's disposable nappy, which, I might as well say, is a ridiculous invention for grown adults. Picture, if you will, my mother lying on the bed, immovable, uncooperative. I unfurled the jumbo nappy and tried with all my might to roll Mum onto the target. My aim was way off and, with the resilience of a brick out-house, she wasn't going anywhere. When I tried to wrangle the nappy beneath her, it started to rip. My frustration was growing as fast as Mum's steely resolve was strengthening.

In a flashback to my old nappy-changing days, I grabbed Mum's two feet and raised them heavenward, hoping her ample derrière might gently lift so I could slide the nappy into position. With a look of absolute horror etched across her face, accompanied by a loud grunt, she performed a swift, full-force, double-legged kick to my guts. I had aroused the beast. My efforts were now being thwarted by a barrage of punches, slaps, schoolgirl pinches and kicks. It was a tantrum of epic proportions.

I began to cry – no, wail – as I fought off the assault, tenaciously sticking to my end goal. Mum appeared completely unmoved (physically and emotionally) by my tears; her empathy obviously shrivelled up somewhere in that shrinking brain of hers.

Opening a crack in the door, I gave a loud SOS call to Ross. He responded with cheetah-like speed, trying hard to appear unfazed by the scene he'd bounded into. I had cobbled the nappy together as best I could under the circumstances, but it was skew-whiff and gaping all over the joint. Ross calmly suggested we try to do it standing up. His soothing presence helped to temporarily stifle Mum's desire to pummel me and, surprisingly, she slid off the bed to a standing position. In a brilliant display of teamwork, we managed to ensure the giant nappy was firmly in place, hopefully ready to do its job through the night. Feeling like I had gone ten rounds in the ring with Danny Green, I pondered the fact that this was definitely not an individual sport.

* * *

With Mum relaxed and quiet on our couch, Molly suggested we play some music for her. Though she was a little preoccupied, stuffing catalogues and tissues into her handbag, eventually Mum began to turn her attention to the sweet sounds emanating from the speakers. With a spark of recognition flashing across her face, she seemed to actually be listening to and enjoying the music.

Drawing on all those years of classical ballet training, Molly began to pirouette and jeté across the room. Mum was mesmerised. There was something quite beautiful in this little scene. Molly beckoned me to join her and, though my moves were far from graceful compared to those of my nimble twenty-two-year-old daughter, I too jumped up to dance. Uninhibited, we twirled and whirled around the lounge room to the soothing harmonies of Air Supply before our delighted audience of one. It was just the therapy I needed and a moment in time I will forever treasure.

A BOTTLE OF RED ...
A BOTTLE OF WHITE

At the time of Mum's diagnosis, her relationship with alcohol was dysfunctional, as I have mentioned. She had been indulging beyond what was normal and causing us to question whether this abuse of alcohol was just a bad habit or, more worryingly, full-blown alcoholism, before we discovered it was in fact a dementia-driven obsession. For this reason, abstinence had been advised and the Leafy Lodge staff had adhered tightly to the doctor's orders for the first few years of Mum's residence there. At every mealtime, the laden drinks cart would glide by, offering a tantalising array of drinks – both alcoholic and non-alcoholic – for the residents to enjoy. Mum would look longingly at the alcoholic beverages but was happy enough to quench her thirst with a ginger beer instead.

I'm not sure when, or what the initial catalyst was, but the staff began allowing Mum to have a glass of vino with her meals. The cork had been popped both literally and metaphorically and now that Jeannie had been reintroduced to the bottle, there was no way of putting the genie back in, so to speak. Spying the dinnertime drinks cart from a mile away, she would home in on the prize, grab her empty cup and give chase. Skolling it in record time, she would then pursue the drinks waiter with the determination of a bull chasing a matador, hoping for a refill. As she downed another plastic cupful of wine, she would grin from ear-to-ear.

The alcohol had an immediate effect on her mood. Initially, she would be jubilant, curiously becoming more lucid and noticeably easier to understand. Unfortunately, that would be followed by a rapid decline into cantankerousness and aggression, leaving us all to wonder whether it was worth it. The tenacity with which Mum tried to procure herself a drop would suggest that, from her point of view anyway, it was. The jury was still out as far as the rest of us were concerned.

During the Catastrophic Fire evacuation, as we assembled at the dining table for our family dinner, it was almost like old times (apart from the fact that Mum chose to remain standing for the first half of the meal). Picking up strands of spaghetti, dangling and chomping on them as she wandered around the table, Mum spied the balsamic vinegar salad dressing sitting on the table. In its fancy glass bottle with the long neck, it could easily have been mistaken for a bottle of red wine. Mum eyed it longingly and would have undoubtedly taken a swig had we not intervened.

We decided to give her a small glass of red, which caused her to immediately take her seat at the head of the table and giggle incessantly. She began to litter her normally incomprehensible babble with identifiable words. It was amazing. We definitely got the general idea of what she was trying to say. She was happy and chatty and making a modicum of sense. Our Spanish friend Maria, a psychology student, had joined us for dinner and was fascinated by this transformation in Mum's behaviour and speech.

Before long, though, as expected, Mum began to get very snappy and uncooperative. Putting her to bed was not a walk in the park that night, I can tell you. Such highs and lows are hard to deal with. Not only is looking after someone with dementia physically demanding, it takes a toll emotionally and mentally as well.

* * *

Once the immediate fire danger had subsided, the Leafy Lodge residents were given the all-clear to return. And all over again, I was racked with guilt. How could I remove her from the refuge of my home, where life carried on as normal and she was surrounded with family who loved and cared for her? How could we give her a taste of normal life and then tear her away from it? How could I take her back to that institution?

My heart was heavy as I parked the car and walked arm-in-arm with Mum to the doors of Leafy Lodge. Would she go in? Would she hate me for it? Would she be full of renewed zeal to leave?

As I typed the first of the security codes required to enter the fortress into the number pad, Mum seemed quite calm. By the time I'd punched in the second code, she was waltzing through the doors without a care in the world – no looking back.

She was immediately embraced by a group of the beautiful staff members, one of whom planted multiple kisses on both her cheeks and, squeezing her tightly, proclaimed, 'Jeannie! We've missed you so much! It's great to have you back!'

Mum was in the thick of an enormous group hug and her expression was one of pure joy as she was welcomed incredibly warmly by those wonderful humans. I felt overwhelmed with gratitude for the love and support she was receiving. This really was her home now. I said a prayer of thanks that my earlier fears had been completely unwarranted.

Mum set out at a cracking pace and strode along a determined trajectory, heading straight for her favourite chair beside the window. If the day's proceedings had been an episode of *Sesame Street*, they would have been brought to us by the letter 'R' and the word 'RELIEF'.

PANDEMIC PANDEMONIUM

The year 2020 will be firmly etched into the memory banks of all who lived through it. As murmurs of this new 'Coronavirus' – a sinister, ultra-contagious affliction; flu-like but deadly – began to spread, we were glued to the news. With its origins traced to the wet markets of far-off Wuhan, it was devastating, but we still felt somewhat safe Down Under.

In a matter of weeks, countries began falling like dominoes, succumbing quickly to contagion. We realised we had a worldwide pandemic on our hands. Italian hospitals swelled past capacity with makeshift wards in town squares; the Spanish were told to work from home. The French closed their tourist attractions. Planes were grounded. Most of Europe was in total lockdown, the streets eerily empty and the health systems stretched to bulging. Cases were multiplying daily at a worrying rate.

Australians were still travelling and going about our daily business while this was happening, but we were now preparing for the worst. When, like a rising tide, the pandemic arrived on the shores of the land 'girt by sea', we stood to attention. Regular updates from the Prime Minister and the premiers were our daily bread, and we watched on in horror as this virus took hold and transformed our lives.

In our household, we had a Year 8 student learning from home, a second-year university student learning from home and a couple of WFH-ers. It was great fun, at first, to feel like part of a real-life hospital drama, scrubbing-in diligently throughout the day, but by bedtime, the old hands were pretty close to shrivelling right up. If not for the technological wonder of video calls, we'd have felt a whole lot more isolated than we did.

We were constantly urged by the relevant authorities to be on the lookout for symptoms: 'If you have a cough, a fever or difficulty breathing, don't muck around. Get yourself to a hospital as soon as possible and get tested.' Everyone was on high alert.

Being a virus that primarily attacked the respiratory system, Coronavirus was most dangerous to the elderly, the frail and the immunocompromised. Leafy Lodge and other facilities like it were full of such individuals – the most vulnerable people around. Not surprisingly, it was only a matter of time before they all went into mandatory lockdown – sadly, not before more than one nursing home had been struck down, a single case leading to an outbreak with fatal results.

The lockdown at Leafy Lodge lasted almost four months and

while they managed to keep the dreaded Corona-lurgy at bay, they kept all of us away too. I missed Mum terribly in that time. It was so hard not knowing how she was. We could call, but the lines were often busy for hours, with other anxious relatives equally hungry for news. A few weeks into lockdown, Leafy Lodge started to offer video calls. What a brilliant idea: a glimpse into the residents' private world.

Seeing Mum's face light up the screen was such a joy. The hint of recognition that registered in her expression when she spotted me was overwhelming. She hadn't forgotten me. Not yet.

While it was great to see her, the video calls were a festival of rhetorical questions:

'How are you, Mum?

'How has your week been?

'What have you been up to?

'Have you been sleeping well?

'What did you have for breakfast?'

I kept on throwing them out there. Mum would usually lose interest around question number three, finding the rest of her surroundings far more compelling to look at than the incessant interrogator on the small screen on her lap.

'Hello?

'Mu-um.

'Yoo-hoo!'

After a couple of agonising minutes of non-comprehension

on my mum's part and zero feedback for me, it just became awkward. It was difficult enough to interact in person; this was very laborious. I may as well have been speaking Swahili. I'd feel embarrassed (and a tad guilty) for wanting to terminate the call so hastily, so would keep jabbering on, doing a tour of the house or tasking my other family members with the quest to engage their nanna or mother-in-law in conversation. My main aim was to soldier on until the staff member would put me out of my misery by saying those words I'd waited so longingly for: 'Well, we might wrap it up there.' Oh, so soon? Secretly, phew.

Ben and Dad fielded their own video calls with Mum. The Leafy Lodge staff said that Ben and his son Will had Mum in stitches with their funny faces. Now, why hadn't I thought of that? But Dad struggled to engage Mum too. It was hard.

As Coronavirus cases began to come under control in New South Wales, Leafy Lodge eased their restrictions for a time. The next step was for limited and controlled visits to take place. Relatives had to book half-hour appointments to see their loved ones. We were met at the exterior door, temperature-checked and made to show our vaccination records. Once our hands had been suitably sanitised, we were escorted to the bedroom for a one-on-one visit.

Our first visit went surprisingly smoothly. Mum and I sat on her bed and together watched a TV doco on animals of the African savanna. She seemed quite content. We rifled through her drawer of miscellaneous lipsticks and make-up. I painted her lips and did her hair and we had fun taking selfies together. With her sunhat at a jaunty angle and her bright red lipstick on, Mum looked more like her old self than she had for a long time.

The next couple of visits did not go so well. All Mum wanted was to leave the room. She became fixated on getting out the door, but I was under strict Coronavirus-safe instructions not to leave the room under any circumstances. Houston, we have a problem. I had no choice but to become a human barricade, my outstretched arms spanning the doorway, for the entire visit. Intent on breaking through said barrier, Mum employed all the kung-fu moves she'd ever learnt from Saturday afternoon re-runs of Bruce Lee movies. Even when she landed a beautiful fly-kick smack in the middle of my shin, my yelp of pain and subsequent tears didn't perturb her one bit or hinder her mission one iota.

I feel a little ashamed to say I was almost relieved when Leafy Lodge went back into lockdown. A second wave of Coronavirus had gripped Victoria and more nursing homes had fallen victim to the ravages of the disease. New South Wales closed its borders and restrictions were re-introduced. Video calls became the main way of 'communicating' with my mother once again.

BACK TO THE FUTURE

Frontotemporal dementia (like Alzheimer's disease, Vascular dementia, and Lewy body dementia) is a degenerative disease. 'Degenerative' is a horrible word. At the time of diagnosis, it seems abstract. The final destination is always the same, yet the road that leads there is winding and laden with detours and potholes you can never fully anticipate. The pace at which someone with dementia declines differs from person to person, so it's not possible to predict its course. There are two promises, however: it will get worse over time and it is irreversible.

Knowing this in theory doesn't adequately prepare you for being an eyewitness to the disease's effects. We, in our family, have all struggled with wanting to know what comes next. If only there were neat stages we could tick off as we went along. When I was pregnant, I loved the book *What to Expect When You are Expecting* by Heidi Murkoff and Sharon Mazel. There is a checklist of what you should be feeling every week, how the pregnancy should be progressing and, as the title suggests, generally what to expect. There are even little pictures. Unfortunately, dementia is not so clear-cut; there is absolutely no way of knowing what to expect.

Advances in the diagnosis and treatment of dementia have been significant in recent years and with more funding being designated for dementia research, hopes for the future are high. As yet though, we are still far from a cure, so from the point of diagnosis, there's no turning back. Brain cells that formerly buzzed with life, held copious filing cabinets chock-full of experiences and memories, silently signalled body parts to move, retained fascinating facts and formulated hypotheses, registered sensations and savoured tastes, created, invented and dreamed, once destroyed, can never return. I long and pray for a day when modern medicine can not only prevent the onset of this monstrous, personality pilfering disease, but can restore what has been lost.

Saint Augustine of Hippo wrote that the mind is a 'vast court; a large and boundless chamber'. Though he wrote this piece way back at the end of the fourth century AD – part of his autobiographical jottings – it sums up beautifully the attributes and abilities of the human mind and what it contains:

And I come to the fields and spacious palaces of my memory, where are the treasures of innumerable images, brought into it from things of all sorts perceived by the senses.

... light, and all colours and forms of bodies by the eyes;

by the ears all sorts of sounds; all smells by the avenue of the nostrils; all tastes by the mouth; and by the sensation of the whole body, what is hard or soft; hot or cold; or rugged; heavy or light; either outwardly or inwardly to the body. All these does that great harbour of the memory receive in her numberless secret and inexpressible windings, to be forthcoming, and brought out at need; each entering in by his own gate, and there laid up ...

When I enter there, I require what I will to be brought forth, and something instantly comes; others must be longer sought after, which are fetched, as it were, out of some inner receptacle; others rush out in troops, and while one thing is desired and required, they start forth ...

For even while I dwell in darkness and silence, in my memory I can produce colours, if I will, and discern between black and white, and what others I will: nor yet do sounds break in and disturb the image drawn in by my eyes, which I am reviewing, though they also are there, lying dormant, and laid up, as it were, apart. For these too I call for, and forthwith they appear. And though my tongue be still, and my throat mute, so can I sing as much as I will; nor do those images of colours, which notwithstanding be there, intrude themselves and interrupt, when another store is called for, which flowed in by the ears. So the other things, piled in and up by the other senses, I recall at my pleasure. Yea, I discern the breath of lilies from violets, though smelling nothing; and I prefer honey to sweet wine, smooth before rugged, at the time neither tasting nor handling, but remembering only.

These things do I within, in that vast court of my memory. For there are present with me, heaven, earth, sea, and whatever I could think on …

Great is this force of memory, excessive great, O my God; a large and boundless chamber! Who ever sounded the bottom thereof?[6]

Without the vast and boundless chamber of our mind, who are we? All our experiences, every single thing we know and have ever known, our history, the opinions we have formed, the ideals we hold, our values, our morals, even our likes and dislikes – these are the things that make us unique individuals. These are the very substance of who we are. Once we have been stripped of all that we are, what is left?

Watching the steady ebb of my mother's personality leaving her was excruciating. Watching the qualities so quintessential to who she was disappear without a trace was painful beyond words. Like a rubbery piece of too-long-chewed chewing gum, the flavour of who she once was had long gone, her essence was depleted.

Though it might seem absurd, the more I visited Mum, the more desperately I missed her.

The glimmer of recognition she may have shown at a well-worn family joke or one of her old ditties eventually drew nothing but a blank.

Every three seconds, someone in the world develops dementia. It's now the number one killer of women in Australia and the second overall leading cause of death in our country. In 2024, it is estimated that more than 421,000 Australians live with dementia.[7] Without a medical breakthrough, the number of people with dementia in this country is expected to increase to more than 812,500 by 2054.[8]

At present, there are many unknowns. Available treatments work at easing or slowing symptoms, but the underlying biological cause for many types of dementia is yet to be discovered. Thankfully, there is much research being undertaken into better ways of diagnosing dementia, identifying its causes and managing treatment. I am confident that one day in the not-so-distant future, there will be a cure.

* * *

So, we plodded on.

One day, I met a lady at the shops who recognised me. She told me that her mum was also a resident of Leafy Lodge. She knew Jeannie as 'the one who babbles all the time – "bah-bah-bah"'. Mum had quite a reputation, it seemed. Sadly, this woman's mother was confined to bed and rarely left her room. She was no longer talking, no longer showing any emotion, consigned to see out her days in a bed on wheels. Barely living.

In the six years Mum was at Leafy Lodge, I'd seen this story play out often. Residents who were once lively and full of energy would suddenly take a nose-dive. They started to look thinner. They stopped walking around. They quietened down. Soon they were being fed by the staff, only able to eat their meals in their beds. They began to sleep for most of the day, and the night.

I would do my own little roll call each time I walked through the doors. Betty is here – check. Nancy is here – check. Edith is here – check. Harry is here – check. Uh-oh. Where is Kevin? I would scan the room for Kevin's familiar smile but it was nowhere to be seen. My fears were confirmed when I received the wretched news that Kevin had shuffled off his mortal coil. I felt sad for his family and realised I'd no longer see them gracing the halls. I couldn't work out if they would feel relieved or devastated, or a little bit of both.

It was a revolving door. When I saw a new face on the scene, I knew they must have taken someone's place. I would tentatively ask the staff, 'Have you lost someone?' It was gut-wrenching to find out someone hadn't made it through the week. I knew then that one day that person would be Mum and the thought of it made me numb.

So, we waited. We'd sit around and wait for the inevitable to happen, for this cruel monster, dementia, to finish the work it had already started by taking away our beautiful Jeannie and leaving only an empty shell of her former self.

EPILOGUE

My daughter, Molly, was studying Art Education at university and had been given the opportunity to go on a study trip to Venice in Italy and the German town of Kassel. She'd planned a couple of weeks either side to gallivant around Europe and have a fabulous holiday. Due to unforeseen circumstances, a couple of friends were forced to pull out at the eleventh hour so, in true Steve Bradbury style, I was lucky enough to become her stand-in travel buddy.

I visited Mum the day before we left and something seemed different. She didn't eat much of her lunch; she seemed very sleepy and even more disinterested in my visit than usual. She didn't look good either, but I couldn't quite put my finger on what was off. I kissed her goodbye and headed off with Molly the next day.

Our first stop was London and, incredibly jet-lagged, we retired early in preparation for a full day of sight-seeing. My phone rang in the middle of the night, which is usually great cause for alarm, but this time I assumed it was just someone who hadn't realised I'd crossed the international dateline and was mid-slumber. I cursed the fact I'd forgotten to slide the button to 'Silent'.

Well, this was no accidental call across the seas. It was the manager of Leafy Lodge, informing me that it might be a good idea to come and see Mum in the next day or two. Apparently, she had become very sleepy over the last couple of days and was now out cold; not in a coma but 'unresponsive'. When I told him a pop-in might be a little tricky, given I was 16,978 kilometres away (give or take a kilometre) and had just embarked on a five-week trip, he assured me that things could turn around. He'd keep me posted. This had happened with Mum once before and she'd rallied and pepped up within twenty-four hours. He was chatting to Ben and Dad too; we'd all be in touch, keeping each other in the proverbial loop.

Over the next day or two, Mum's condition worsened. Because we'd ticked the 'Do not resuscitate' box on the *Advanced Care Directives* plan, it was decided that she would remain at Leafy Lodge, in the care of those she knew.

Ben called with the devastating news from the doctor that Mum probably wouldn't last out the week. I really didn't know what to do. Being so far away, I was scared Mum would die while I was mid-air and I'd miss out on seeing her for one last cuddle. Worse still, she'd breathe her last while I was travelling and I'd find out two days later. Should I stay where I was until I heard news of Mum's passing, or should I come home and wait for her to die? She was still unconscious and wouldn't wake up. It was impossible to know what to do.

I prayed a lot.

After much deliberation, it was decided that I'd wait until Mum had passed away and then come straight home to make plans for the funeral. Molly would stay and continue the trip. She hadn't been keen on travelling alone – hence my late inclusion in the plans – but this study tour was such a great opportunity. We would Zoom her in for the funeral. Ben and Dad would together bear the brunt of the last couple of days of Mum's life without me, which I felt conflicted about. They assured me this was a good plan – the best we could do in the circumstances.

A day later, while Molly and I sat in the main street of Dover, right next to a big stone church, built in 1203, it struck me that this building had stood proudly on the same corner for over 800 years, robust and unchanging. What a contrast to the fragility of human life.

While Molly sorted out our bus route, I met the delightful ninety-five-year-old Elsie, who had recently lost her husband to dementia and was about to go on a cruise to Portugal that her daughter had booked for them, hoping to cheer her up. She patted me on the leg and told me she was a realist and doubted any cruise would lift her mood. She'd spent years caring for her dear husband, watching him deteriorate as his brain retreated. When I told her about Mum, a bridge of understanding formed between us and we both had a cry there on the park bench.

Molly and I dined on chips and cheddar at the historic Coast Guard Pub on the bay, with a clear view of France across the water. Then we started on the long walk back up the hill towards Dover's famous white cliffs. As we dodged gigantic bumble bees and ate wild blackberries from along the sides of the path, we felt like we were in an episode of *Escape to the Country*. All the houses had names like 'Badger Walk' and 'Avonsea'. Just as we were cresting the hill, Ben called to tell me the dreadful news I'd been waiting for: our beautiful mum had passed away.

I had wondered over these past years how the news would make me feel. Obviously, the grieving process had started long before now and so I was surprised by how devastated I felt. Ben aptly described the feeling of living with someone suffering from dementia as 'reading a book three-quarters of the way through'. We had known the book would end in a certain way; now, here was the final chapter.

Perhaps during the course of Mum's dementia, I had avoided dwelling too much on the past and had tried to focus on the present, working on ways to cope with the 'new' Mum and love her the way she was. Once she was gone, all the memories came gushing back and I allowed myself to remember her as she was before dementia. The loss felt immense.

Ben sent me a photo of Mum lying in her Leafy Lodge room,

drained of life and colour. It was confronting and excruciatingly sad. We had a video call; he let me see her and be there in the room with them both. Dad, Ross and Julie were on their way. I am so grateful Ben was there with Mum when she breathed her last.

So, on we walked, Molly and I, across the breathtakingly stunning and unique Dover coastline, me bawling and Molly a great comfort. We walked, cried and talked for a whopping five and a half hours and were relieved when we finally reached the town of Dover. It was getting dark and there were only a few trains going back to London after the sun went down. We had a deadline! My phone battery was fading fast and Molly had no wi-fi, so we couldn't really work out where we were going. We came to the Dover Visitor's Centre, a beacon of hope for our weary legs and heavy hearts, but alas, it was closed. Molly had suggested we ask a 'nice stranger' for a lift earlier in the day, to which I'd said, 'Hitchhiking? No way! Too dangerous.' Now, after almost six hours of trekking in the relentless sun and with apparently still a long way to go, I'd have been happy to be strapped to someone's roof racks.

On our way down the steps into the town, we met a lovely Englishman called Peter. He was probably about ten years older than me but fit as a fiddle. You could crack nuts on his calf muscles. We explained our dilemma and the fact that our somewhat puffy eyes were less to do with being lost and more to do with the news I'd just received about my mother. His eyes filled with tears as he explained that his own father had battled with dementia for the past five years and had passed away during the lockdowns of the pandemic a year before. He too had been unable to be with his parent when he had died. He knew exactly how I felt. What a godsend he was. We hugged and, with a hearty 'Follow me! I'll get you there on time', he beckoned his two very bedraggled travelling companions onwards and upwards, vowing to get us on the last train to London.

APPENDIX

Dementia is not a specific disease. It is an umbrella term used to describe a number of disorders characterised by symptoms affecting memory, behaviour and the ability to interact with others and perform normal, everyday tasks. Caused by damage to nerve cells in various areas of the brain, brain function is affected as cells die and parts of the brain shrink and cease to perform the tasks they were designed for.

It has been eye-opening to learn that many families of dementia sufferers are told by medical professionals that their loved ones are suffering from 'dementia', with no explanation of the type of dementia they have. Different types of dementia will produce different symptoms in individuals, depending on which area of the brain the damage has occurred.

The main types of dementia are Alzheimer's disease, vascular dementia, Lewy body disease, frontotemporal lobar degeneration (FTLD), Huntington's disease, alcohol-related dementia (Korsakoff syndrome) and Creutzfeldt-Jakob disease. Each has its own symptoms and causes but there are many similarities between the different types as well.

Here is a brief rundown of each of the main types:

Alzheimer's disease
Alzheimer's disease is the most common form of dementia, accounting for around 70 per cent of all dementia cases. Primarily affecting memory, Alzheimer's disease was named after Dr Alois Alzheimer, who was the first to record a case, in 1907.

Short-term memory loss is usually the first symptom of Alzheimer's disease. It typically strikes after the age of sixty-five but is more common in those over eighty-five, with three in ten people in that age bracket affected.

Abnormal proteins – 'tangles' inside the brain cells and 'plaques' outside the brain cells – build up in the brain, interrupting communication between brain cells, which leads to the eventual shrinkage of the brain and cessation of function.

Eventually, as Alzheimer's progresses, long-term memory is also lost, and many areas of behaviour are affected. Other symptoms include vagueness in everyday conversation, general loss of enthusiasm, inability to follow or process instructions, emotional unpredictability, forgetting places and people (including loved ones) and a decline in social skills.

Vascular dementia
Vascular dementia results from reduced or diminished blood flow to the blood vessels in the brain, causing damage to the brain. It is the second most common form of dementia.

It can result from stroke, high blood pressure, raised cholesterol, heart valve infection or general blood vessel conditions. There are two main types of vascular dementia: multi-infarct dementia and Binswanger's disease (also known as subcortical vascular dementia).

Multi-infarct dementia's symptoms can develop gradually, often after a number of strokes. Damage to the cortex of the brain, where learning, language and memory reside, may result in mood swings, severe depression or the onset of epilepsy.

Binswanger's disease is caused by elevated blood pressure and the resulting thickening of the arteries and reduced blood flow. Symptoms include loss of the ability to walk and loss of bladder control. Mood swings and lethargy are also common symptoms.

Smoking, high blood pressure, high cholesterol, abnormal heart rhythms and diabetes can all lead to stroke, which can lead to vascular dementia. While there is no cure for vascular dementia, many steps can be taken to reduce the risk of stroke, such as monitoring sugar and cholesterol intake, not smoking and keeping blood pressure within a normal range.

People suffering from vascular dementia may also have other forms of dementia, like Alzheimer's disease.

Frontotemporal dementia (FTD/FTLD)

Also known as frontotemporal lobar degeneration, behavioural-variant dementia and Pick's disease, frontotemporal dementia was first discovered by Arnold Pick 100 years ago. It is another common type of dementia.

Its onset is typically earlier than that of Alzheimer's disease, with cases in individuals in their fifties, sixties and even as young as thirties.

Brain cells in the frontal and/or temporal lobes are initially affected. The left and right lobes at the front of the brain (frontal) are responsible for social behaviour, mood, attention span, judgement, planning and self-control. Though short-term memory can be affected, memory loss isn't always a symptom, especially in the early stages. Changes to behaviour and personality are usually the first signs of this type of dementia, making it difficult to diagnose.

Other symptoms are loss of emotional warmth and empathy, apathy and lack of motivation, lack of social interaction, loss of inhibition and tact, difficulty in planning, reasoning and organisation, a decline in self-care and hygiene, craving sweet foods, overeating or indulging, and an inability to adapt or be flexible, which comes across as obstinance or selfishness. As the disease progresses, obsessive behaviours can also be displayed.

The temporal lobes of the brain determine what we see and hear and how we understand things. If there is damage to the temporal lobes, language can be impaired and/or eventually lost. A person may have trouble recognising or naming an object and could have difficulty in expressing themselves.

There are two types of FTD in which language is affected: progressive non-fluent aphasia and semantic dementia. In progressive non-fluent aphasia, speech becomes difficult and may be punctuated with wrong words or wrong grammar, whereas semantic dementia sufferers gradually lose their vocabulary and knowledge of words. Speech will continue to become vague and may disappear altogether, and reading and writing skills may also be affected.

Lewy body disease
Caused by the breakdown and eventual death of the nerve cells in the brain, Lewy body disease is named after the abnormal spherical structures that develop inside nerve cells, called Lewy bodies. German doctor, Friedric Heinrich Lewy, discovered these protein deposits, hence the name.

There is no known cause for this type of dementia and no identifying risk factors.

Around 10 per cent of all dementia patients suffer from Lewy body disease, also called Diffuse Lewy body disease. Symptoms mimic those of Parkinson's disease – slow movements, unsteady gait, clumsiness, a high propensity for falls and tremors – making distinguishing between the two difficult at times. It can also be confused with Alzheimer's disease, sharing many symptoms, such as difficulties with concentration and memory, extreme confusion and lack of facial expression.

Hallucinations and delusions are often common for those suffering from Lewy body dementia. Rapid fluctuations in mental state can also occur, where one minute the person is lucid and the next, they are disoriented, confused or bewildered. Sleeping, lethargy and staring spells are also symptoms of Lewy body disease.

REFERENCES AND RESOURCES

AFTDA (Australian Fronto-Temporal Dementia Association) (www.theaftd.org.au)

Alzheimer's Disease International, USA (alzint.org)

Alzheimer's Research Australia, in particular see the page '10 Signs'. (https://alzheimersresearch.org.au/alzheimers/10-signs/)

Dementia Australia (www.dementia.org.au)

FDT (Fronto-Temporal Dementia) Talk, UK, see their factsheets. (www.ftdtalk.org/factsheets/)

National Dementia Helpline: 1800 100 500

Neura, an independent, not-for-profit, medical research institute dedicated to improving the lives of people living with brain and nervous system disorders. (www.neura.edu.au)

Rare Dementia Support, UK (www.raredementiasupport.org)

ENDNOTES

1   Førsund, L.H., Grov, E.K., *et al.*, 'The experience of lived space in persons with dementia: a systematic meta-synthesis'. *BMC Geriatrics*. 18(1), 1 February 2018. See also: Olsen, C., Pedersen, I., Bergland, A. *et al.*, 'Differences in quality of life in home-dwelling persons and nursing home residents with dementia – a cross-sectional study'. *BMC Geriatrics,* 16(137), 11 July 2016.

2   1 Samuel 16:7, Holy Bible (NIV).

3   Baird, A., Garrido, S., & Tamplin, J., *Music and Dementia: From Cognition to Therapy.* Oxford University Press, 2019.

4   Garner, Helen, *Everywhere I Look*, Text Publishing Company, 2016. This is a collection of Garner's essays and includes an essay about her mother, 'Dreams of Her Real Self'.

5   Fatuzzo, I., Niccolini, G. F., *et al.*, 'Neurons, nose, and neurodegenerative diseases: olfactory function and cognitive impairment'. *International Journal of Molecular Sciences*, 24(3), 2023.

6   *Augustine Confessions* 10.8-12 397-400 AD. From Saint Augustine of Hippo's autobiographical work. He wrote it in Latin, when in his early 40s and his memory was still sharp.

7   Institute of Health and Welfare, 'Dementia in Australia', *AIHW*, Australian Government, 2022.

8   *Alzheimer's Disease: Facts & Figures.* Reviewed by Sharyn Rossi PhD, Alzheimer's Disease Research, Bright Focus Foundation, brightfocus.org. Updated April 2024.

ACKNOWLEDGEMENTS

It goes without saying that I'd like to thank my mum, Jeannie Somerville. Thanks, Mum, for loving me so fiercely and completely and for absolutely all the love and light you have injected into my life. I miss you beyond belief.

Thank you to all my early readers and encouragers, including Martyn and Julie Toole, Ellen Jenkinson, Michelle Madder, Keryn Gallagher and my lovely book club girls, Jennie Rothwell, Barbara Clarke, Heidi Brunker, Jacquie Martin, Kate Crouch, Jenny Nagel, Lindy Green, Jenny Andresen, Toni Konijn and Sue Jacobs. Thanks for your early feedback and unwaveringly enthusiastic support of my writing.

Great thanks also to Ingrid Ohlsson for giving me a chance and for pointing me in the right direction.

Thanks to Liz Seymour for the beautiful cover design, really capturing in pictures what I wanted to convey in my book and for your expertise in making my book look good.

Thanks to Nicole Webb for guidance in how to get my book out into the world, your experience has been much appreciated.

Bernadette Foley, you have been such a warm and wonderful guiding light, a source of inspiration and mentor. I couldn't have done this without you. Thank you!

All the love in the world and thanks go to my brother Ben Somerville, his wife Julie Somerville, their gorgeous offspring Sophie, Will and Emily and my dad Tony Somerville, who have all played supporting actor roles in this story we have shared together. Thanks for allowing me to tell the story and for all your love and support.

I am eternally grateful for my own family and their love – my darling husband Ross and my beautiful kids Sam, Molly, Toby and Maisy. Thanks for loving me unconditionally and for your patience with my writing (most of the time!). I love you all to bits.

Thanks also to my wonderful blog readers – the faithful stalwarts who tune in to read about all our adventures and encourage me to continue with my passion to write. Lisa Bale, Debbie Peters, I'm looking at you! All my readers' comments and kind words have spurred me on to continue to write and have put a spring in my step. Thank you!

The special folk who looked after and nurtured Mum in care – Rachel, Jo, Zeta, Hilda, Jackie and all the incredibly patient and selfless staff. Thanks for being so good at your jobs and for bringing the smile back to Mum's face.

Lastly but certainly not least, I'd like to thank my Almighty God, from whom all good things come. Thanks for continuing to guide me and lead me in my life, for knowing me, giving me meaning and loving me unconditionally.

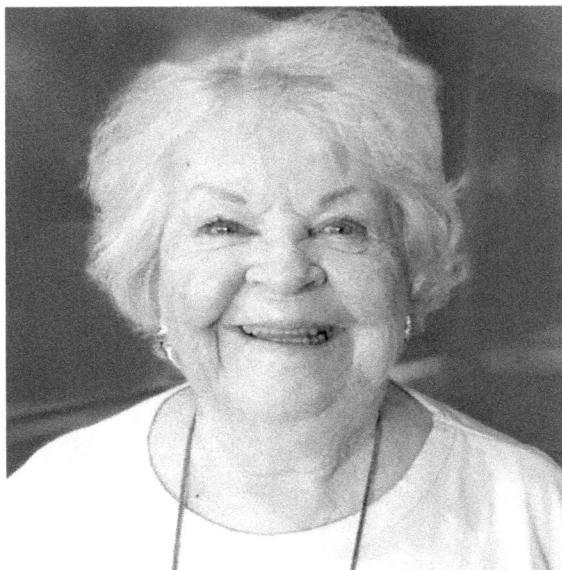

Jeannie Margaret Somerville

27 October 1941 – 9 August 2022